LEARNING TO HEAL

One Woman's Journey Through Medicine

Liz Casper

Available as an ebook

ISBN 978-1-968640-60-6 (paperback)

ISBN 978-1-968640-61-3 (hardcover)

Publify Publishing

Lampasas, TX 76550

contact@publifypublishing.com

LizCasper.com

Dedication

I dedicate this book to all the medical doctors in my family: those who have earned this title before me and those who have followed after me. And I salute all physicians who have survived and thrived in one of the oldest and most noble of professions.

Author's Note and Disclaimer

This book chronicles some of my experiences in medicine as I learned how to heal others and myself. These stories highlight my experiences during medical school, residency training, as a physician in private practice, and as a patient myself.

If you are suffering from any medical condition or illness, please seek the appropriate medical attention before beginning, changing, or ending any regimen of medicine, nutrition, or supplements.

I do not intend this book to replace the advice of physicians or health care practitioners; nor am I intending to diagnose or prescribe treatment for any illness or disorder. What is written is my personal story only. Names have been changed to comply with privacy laws.

I hope you find these stories of interest and perhaps helpful.

Contents

Prologue

I wrote this book, *Learning to Heal*, for anyone who wants to learn more about medicine and the pursuit of a medical doctorate. I aim to give perspective and insight into the path to becoming an allopathic physician, and the challenges and rewards for doing so.

Becoming a medical doctor is a daunting endeavor, even for the most intellectually gifted applicants. Medical school is a four-year, post-graduate doctorate, followed by three to seven or more years of additional training in your chosen specialty. It is highly competitive with a rigorous curriculum, culminating in a medical doctorate (M.D.) degree.

Presently, in the United States, there are approximately 160 accredited institutions that train budding medical doctors. The acceptance rate each year is dismal, with many schools accepting 10% or less of their applicants. Competition is fierce, and many highly qualified students have to apply year after year to gain acceptance.

To become a medical student, you must have great grades from college with a minimum requirement of science: physics, organic chemistry, physical chemistry, and biology. Then, you must "ace" the Medical College Admission Test (MCATs), a comprehensive, day-long test, which confers your mastery of the basic science subject matter to enter medical school.

I had started my undergraduate college work at an East Coast, Ivy League school, but I ended up finishing my last three years of college on the West Coast. I received a bachelor's degree in science, with a major in art, a combination that suited me perfectly. I pursued art with a passion and seriously considered it as a future career. But all that changed when my art thesis advisor suggested I take an anatomy course to better hone my drawing skills of the human body, which still suck to this day.

On my first day of anatomy in college, I had a lightbulb moment, and I knew I had found my calling: medicine. I loved everything about what I was learning in anatomy and prepared myself for the rigors of medical school. I switched most of my art classes for science courses and applied to one medical school. If accepted, I would be a fourth-generation physician in my family, and the first female in my lineage to be one.

Before starting medical school, I had little to reference for what lay ahead for me. Although I hailed from a medical family, I had no intention for the first 26 years of my life to carry on the family tradition. In my family, medicine was reserved for men. My father, a trauma surgeon, was rarely home, and certainly never encouraged me to pursue medicine. Women in my family were artists, teachers, or nurses. Not doctors. Undeterred and without any family encouragement, I forged ahead.

The first two years of medical school are spent primarily in the classroom, listening to one didactic session after another, focused on foundational sciences like anatomy and physiology, biochemistry, and pharmacology. The third and fourth years are primarily focused on clinical skills, with month-long rotations in primary care and subspecialties. Clinical time is spent both in the hospital and in outpatient clinics.

The hours are long, the work is generally thankless, and one's commitment to becoming a physician is frequently challenged. Many call the four years of medical school a "weeding out" phase, and some students do indeed drop out every year due to the overwhelming demands that challenge the body, mind, and soul.

I came into medicine later in life and was called a "non-traditional student" due to my advanced age: I began medical school at the ripe, old age of 27, in the early 1990s. My entering class at the university program was the first time where the women in the program outnumbered the men, 51:49. But as I quickly learned, medicine was still very much a "boy's club" at that time.

Additionally, there was no legal limit to the number of hours per week that one could be asked to work as a medical student, oftentimes exceeding 100 hours per week, all while paying for the privilege to do so for four years. The study of medicine is rigorous, intentionally so, and the schedule grueling. Undeterred, I excitedly entered my program.

When I arrived in the Ivory Halls on my first day of medical school, I literally had to pinch myself. It was hard to believe that just a few short months ago, 18 to be exact, I had pivoted to pre-med. I had applied to only one medical school with an acceptance rate below 5%, and I was fortunate to be accepted the first year I applied. Here I was, ready to attend class, with no idea of what awaited me. I was married, but childless, when I entered the world of medicine.

Chapter 1
Adventures in Anatomy

My first class on my first day of medical school was Anatomy, albeit from a very different perspective as a doctor-to-be rather than as an undergraduate student. I walked into the vast lecture hall and took my seat in the front row, not realizing this would assign me the label of a "goodie two-shoes," and would ostracize me from my much-cooler and younger peers.

Later, I found out that the supposed smartest people in the class - the future neurosurgeons and plastic surgeons of the world - occupied the last row of seats at the back of the auditorium. Clearly, I had announced my IQ, or lack thereof, by choosing the front row. I had always picked the front row of lecture halls due to my impaired distance vision and my keen auditory learning abilities. It had never occurred to me before that choosing a seat in an auditorium could be so defining. Undeterred, I sat in the front row for two years.

Anatomy and Physiology took up a great deal of our time in the first year of medical school. We would learn by dissecting a human body on both a macro- and microscopic level. Every session in the cadaver lab was preceded by a didactic lecture carefully reviewing the day's planned dissection. After class, we would change into our "cadaver scrubs," which granted us access to the cadaver lab.

The large cadaver lab room was located in the basement of the university. It was filled with rows and rows of metal tables housing dead bodies. Sinks and medical supplies for dissection lined the walls of the lab. It was clean, but not sterile, and brightly lit with fluorescent lights. The dissection of a human body was tightly controlled by the professor and the lecture topic that preceded the time in the lab. We were told not to stray from the specific plan for the dissection or face serious consequences.

After our first anatomy lecture, we headed to the cadaver lab where we were randomly assigned a dead body with three other of our classmates. As I entered the lab, a waft of formaldehyde-laden air assaulted my senses, and I nearly turned around and walked out, not sure I could proceed. The smell of a preserved dead body is hard to describe and is anything but pleasant. Row after row of plastic-encased dead bodies awaited to educate us.

I slowly approached my assigned table with trepidation, knowing I would imminently be seeing a preserved, dead body. The thick, black plastic body bag was sealed with a zipper closure that we would use to protect our charge between our thrice-weekly lab sessions. Each body would be our constant companion for the rest of the year, and taking care of our "patient instructor" was a very important part of our learning. We were expected to conduct ourselves as professionals in the lab at all times.

When you are assigned a body (a bag, really), you don't know who will greet you when you reveal the contents. Body donation for medical science in the early 1990s was the only way to learn anatomy firsthand. Technological and medical advancements in the cadaver lab had not kept pace with other innovations, and real human bodies, not computer simulations, were the norm at that time. To be honest, I don't believe a computer model could ever replace the learning from a once-live human. Medical schools and medical science relied on the generous donations of the human body to the cause.

Most of the desired bodies for medical school student dissections were those people who had lived a "good life," dying from old age or something straightforward like cancer or a heart attack. Bodies that had suffered significant or disfiguring trauma were not usually selected in the cadaver lab. The goal was for us students to determine the cause of death after careful dissection, rather than simply diagnosing an obvious automobile accident or gun injury. Most of the bodies in the lab were elderly, and no body was accepted in the lab if they had donated any of their organs.

After locating my body, I stood beside the body on the table and greeted my three classmates. A total of four students per cadaver was a luxury of sorts, as many medical schools at that time assigned six students per body, in an attempt to save money. In my undergraduate anatomy course, we had only one body to dissect for 30 students, so this was quite different and much more intimate. With only four of us working on our body, we were assured lots of individual "table time" with our charge.

All cadavers at that time were zipped up in thick, black plastic bags to keep the formaldehyde stench to a minimum. It also kept the body hydrated and preserved as much as possible for the months-long dissection. The bodies in the lab emitted a pungent smell, made worse over the weeks and months as we carefully dissected the person from head to toe. After each session, we would carefully put the body back together as best we could before zipping it back up in the body bag. After each week in the lab, the body was a bit more dried out and less useful to those of us dissecting it. We were racing against time and dehydration.

As we four medical students surrounded the metal table and body bag, we introduced ourselves. Hose, a short, stout Hispanic man, was a former pharmacist and an "older" student like me. He had found the job of being a pharmacist far too restrictive for his curious mind and was thrilled to be in medical school. Bobby, another tablemate, was fresh out of college and displayed a youthful disrespect for our activities in the lab. He often caused trouble at our table with his antics, and we did our best to squelch his youthful hubris. *Probably a future orthopedist,* I thought to myself.

John, our fourth, was also newly out of college, but much more serious than Bobby. He had completed his college at an Ivy League school, and he definitely took his role in the lab seriously, as did I. The four of us introduced ourselves to each other and flipped a coin for who would have the pleasure of unzipping the body bag for the first time.

Hose won the coin flip, or lost as the case may be, and took a deep breath in as he moved to the head of the table and gingerly unzipped the black plastic. The four of us peered our heads over the table and gasped as he pulled back the cover to reveal an elderly woman who appeared to have died *very* recently. We glanced around at the other tables nearby and noticed that our body was much more hydrated and "fresh" than many others in the lab. Half joking, we checked her skin to make sure she wasn't still warm. Just then, our professor arrived at our table and exclaimed to us, "You guys are lucky! You got a fresh body!" To which Bobby replied, "Let's call her 'Juicy Lucy!

Juicy Lucy was our formal anatomy instructor and constant companion during our first year of medical school. It may sound strange, but the four of us really bonded over our work on Lucy. It never escaped me that she gave her remaining flesh to us so that we could have the privilege to become doctors. We learned, after many months of careful dissection, that Lucy had died of uterine cancer, had heart disease, and her brain looked like Swiss cheese, indicating severe dementia of some type.

Our professor told us we were fortunate to have such a diseased corpse, for learning purposes, of course. The simple car accident of a young, healthy person is much more of a "vanilla" dissection, she said. I always found that reference to be a bit odd. For the most part, the dissections were intense but uneventful. We spent hours bent over the table, carefully picking Lucy apart, one organ system at a time. Shenanigans in the lab were discouraged, and most of us worked diligently and quietly on our assigned dissections.

Occasionally, one of the bodies in the lab would present with an unusual or unique finding, which usually meant we would all leave our body to take a first-hand look at the disease or anomaly. Additionally, we were able to view interesting maladies through a projected microscope. Cancer, infections, heart disease, Alzheimer's, and more were seen from a macro- and microscopic perspective, and the learning was invaluable in beginning to understand the human body.

One day, toward the end of our time with Lucy, Hose was dissecting the gallbladder and bile duct. Frustrated with what appeared to be a clog, he "went off script" and located a syringe with saline and began to flush the duct. Across the table, Bobby watched in fascination as Hose handled the issue with aplomb. The only problem was that when Hose flushed the duct, Lucy's bile shot out of her body and landed directly into Bobby's open mouth. John, Hose, and I could hardly contain our laughter as Bobby ran out of the lab, spitting and sputtering. Fortunately, these types of events were very rare in the anatomy lab.

Our final stint with Juicy Lucy - who wasn't juicy anymore at that point - came on the last day of anatomy class as we neared the end of our first year of medical school. Hose, Bobby, John, and I stood around the table and each of us thanked her for donating her body to science, and for our learning at her expense. Before we left the lab at the end of the year, we prepared Lucy's completely dissected, dried-out body for cremation, and zipped up the body bag for the last time.

Chapter 2
Dean Rude

The first two years of medical school are spent predominantly in the classroom and labs. The third and fourth years are spent on clinical rotations in a hospital, the VA, or outpatient clinics. Learning in medical school has been likened to drinking water from a fire hose. The information comes at you fast and furiously, but you realize you are only capable of handling a few sips at a time. The rest of the learning experience, and cementing of what you've crammed into your brain, will come over the ensuing months, years, and decades.

Most of the time, the best you can hope for is to learn enough to get by in medical school, and most importantly, to not cause harm. "First Do No Harm," an oath I would ultimately take as a physician, was always at the back of my mind. To be a competent physician, you must commit yourself to lifelong learning.

It is very easy to have a love-hate relationship with medical school and medicine in general. The information you are asked to learn is overwhelming, and medicine changes constantly. Often, the things you learned last year can either be outdated or will have improved or changed protocols put in place today. In addition, with the advent of the internet, patients come to their doctor appointments armed with information from Dr. Google. This can enhance, complicate, or even derail the care you had planned for your patient.

Dr. Google might also negate the information you just crammed into your brain, possibly an algorithm or treatment plan in opposition to your patient's self-diagnosis and own ideas for treatment. This can make it seem at times that the medical provider and the patient are at odds with each other, causing tension between patient and physician, potentially impacting care and outcomes. Medicine is a complex career, full of wonderful and innumerable benefits associated with helping people. But the stress, fatigue, and overwhelm can cause burnout, or even worse. Doctors have one of the highest suicide rates of all professions.

In my second year of medical school at the age of 28, and while sitting in an OBGYN lecture, I learned that if you give birth to your first child by age 30, your lifetime risk of breast cancer plummets. Given that I was already married and my husband and I had talked about having children, I decided that I needed to get pregnant - right away - to give birth by the age-30 cutoff deadline.

That same day, I came home from school and had "the talk" with my husband. What resulted was a pregnancy in short order. I had never been pregnant before, so I had little idea of what to expect. I decided in the end to have both of my children during medical school. To have a proper maternity leave with each of my children, I wanted to extend my education by one year. This was a novel idea at the time, and one that had yet to be challenged in my institution.

Up to that point, if a female student elected to have a child during medical school, something that was openly frowned upon, they would be granted only a two-week leave from school with their newborn child. I knew this was not enough time for me as the mother of an infant.

To extend my schooling by a year, I had to meet with one of the Deans of Students and plead my case. The dean was an old man who was overdue to retire, but it was assumed by the students that he was milking his position for every last year of tenure and dollar that he could. None of the students liked him, and we all generally avoided him, save for the occasional lectures he would provide to us in his area of specialty.

One day, after summoning up the courage, I approached the Dean's office without an appointment. I had mild anxiety about my mission as I had no idea how he was going to receive my request. I took the stairs to the top of one of the research buildings on campus and walked down the long, dark corridor. The building appeared empty except for the end of the hall on the right, where there was light shining through an open door. The air smelled musty and heavy as I walked down the hall.

As I approached the open door, I could hear Dr. Dean talking on the phone with what must have been one of his golfing buddies. He was laughing and talking excitedly about their next planned golf trip to Scotland. I cleared my throat loudly so that he would hear me approaching, but he either didn't hear me or ignored me. I sat down on an old, cane chair in an adjacent room lined with old, smelly books and medical relics, and waited for ten minutes until he finished his call.

"Oh, hello," Dr. Dean said in a surprised tone as he exited his office into his library, "I didn't know you were waiting. Do you have an appointment with me?" He appeared concerned that I might have heard his conversation.

"Hello, Dr. Dean, my name is Liz Casper," I said as I stood to shake his hand. "I'm a second-year medical student, and no, I don't have an appointment," I stated. "Do you have a minute?" I asked.

"How can I help you?" he asked as he looked intently at me and squinted his eyes.

I took a deep breath and told him my story. I shared with him my hope to extend my four years of medical school into five so that I could spend more time with my future infant children. As I shared more about my desired plan, his face lost all traces of a smile, and a deeply concerned look came over him.

"Let me get this straight. You want to take an extra year of medical school so that you can have *children*?" he asked incredulously as his voice became louder.

"Yes, sir, I would like to make it through medical school in five years, rather than four, so that I may have more time on maternity leave with my future children," I replied. I didn't dare divulge to him that I was already pregnant. *Maybe we should have had this conversation before I became pregnant?* I wondered to myself. I started to feel very uncomfortable and vulnerable.

At that point, Dr. Dean started to look impatient and pissed off. He checked his watch, leaned toward me, lowered his voice, and spoke to me in a near whisper.

"Young lady," he started, "You are taking up the rightful place of a man in this institution. You don't belong here," he finished.

I couldn't believe what I was hearing. *Did he really just say that?* I asked myself. The year was 1994, and I was sure that women had made far more progress than this in the medical workforce. Screw the school! I was going to take an extra year when I was *paying* for the privilege of being there! And, to take this extra year, I would have to pay for that additional year of medical school. *This is unbelievable!* I said to myself.

Undeterred, and with as much confidence as I could muster, I continued with my reason for visiting. I stepped back from Dr. Dean and his bad, cigar breath, and asked, "So, is that a 'Yes'"?

"I'll let you know. We have never had this issue present itself before, so I will have to speak with the other deans. Don't get your hopes up," he shot back as he turned on his heel and disappeared back into his office. He shut the door behind him, leaving me all alone in his musty library. *I guess this conversation is finished,* I thought to myself as I turned around and left the room.

Women in medicine who want to have children face significant challenges due to the rigors of medical school and residency. Women report insufficient time for family planning or recovery post-delivery. Many programs lack formal policies on family leave, relegating women to negotiate maternity leave informally and individually with their institution, as I had to.

Having children can delay, or even derail, a woman in medical training, leading to perceptions of reduced commitment or lower competency. Women in medicine who want to have a family face stigma and bias as colleagues may perceive them as less dedicated to medicine, which can lead to fewer career opportunities. A 2018 study in the *Journal of the American Medical Association (JAMA)* found 60% of female resident physicians reported delaying pregnancy due to training demands.

I had to wait over a month for the school's decision, but in the end, I did end up being allowed to take the additional year to spend more time with my infant children. After I set the precedent at the university, three female medical students a year behind me did the same thing. *Perhaps having children can be compatible with being a doctor?* I wondered.

Dr. Dean died not too long after my interaction with him. Couldn't have happened to a nicer guy. I'm sure he would roll over in his grave at the thought that a woman might replace him as dean one day.

Chapter 3
Food as Medicine

Early in my third year of medical school, and before I became obviously pregnant, I was assigned to a month-long rotation in an outpatient family practice clinic. The clinic was exceptionally busy and was led by a married pair of physicians, Drs. X and Y. These two were affectionately known as "hippies" and were respected for their unorthodox approach to certain illnesses. It was hard to get assigned to their clinic because the rotation was so popular. I was excited for the opportunity to have an outpatient experience in the community with them, rather than a hospital system.

In the early 1990s, family practice was a specialty encompassing the care of adults, children, and pregnant women. It was considered one of the most difficult specialties due to the depth and breadth of information you were expected to know. Essentially three specialties in one medical career: OBGYN, internal medicine (a doctor for adults), and pediatrics. All those specialties require only three years of residency training after medical school. Family medicine at that time attracted a highly intelligent and committed physician who could handle the wide variety of patients.

I arrived early for my first day in the family practice clinic. I entered the office through the front door, patient entrance, and marveled at the full waiting room. Patients of all ages and stages of life filled the chairs. I waited in line behind patients checking in at the reception desk, and once it was my turn, I addressed the receptionist.

"Hi, my name is Liz. I am starting my rotation here today."

"Hi Liz, nice to meet you. Enter through this door and you will see the breakroom on your right," the receptionist answered as she gestured to a door to the back office labeled "private." I found the break room and squeezed my lunch in the overflowing employee fridge before taking a seat to wait for further instructions.

A few minutes later, a medical assistant in scrubs came into the room and introduced herself. "Hi, you must be Liz. I'm Lorraine, Dr. X's medical assistant. Are you ready for a busy day?" she asked cheerily and with a bright smile.

"Ready!" I replied enthusiastically as I stood up from my chair.

"Follow me," she replied as she turned around and left the breakroom.

I followed Lorraine as we weaved ourselves through the labyrinth of halls and exam rooms in the big clinic. As we approached exam room #7, Dr. X emerged and handed a paper patient chart to Lorraine. She quickly gave her some instructions for her to complete for the patient still in the room.

Lorraine took the paperwork from her and said, "Dr. X, this is Liz, our medical student this month."

"Hi Liz! We are thrilled to have you with us. Over the next month, you will be working with both my husband, Dr. Y, and me. Today you and I are together. Follow me," she said as she started walking down the hall toward another exam room.

Dr. X did indeed look like a hippie. She was wearing a long maxi dress in vibrant colors, a vest with fringe, and Birkenstocks with socks, out of character for most physicians at the time. She and her husband had also decided to forego wearing the white "doctor coat" in their clinic in an attempt to be more relatable to their patients. She was middle-aged, generally attractive, and full of energy.

I followed Dr. X down the hall toward another exam room, #9. She stopped before entering the room and pulled the paper chart from the cubby, and quickly reviewed it. As she flipped through a few chart notes, lab results, and vaccination records, she began to introduce me to the patient and his reason for being at the clinic that day.

"Liz, we are going to see Bobby now. He has been our patient since I delivered him seven years ago. His parents are worried that he might have Attention-Deficit/Hyperactivity Disorder (ADHD). We are going to discuss this today," she finished as she reached for the door handle.

"Knock, knock," Dr. X said quietly as she opened the door, instead of actually knocking. "Hi, Mom. Hi Bobby! I have a guest with us today, Liz, who's a student doctor." I smiled and shook hands with Bobby's mother.

We all took our place in the exam room with Bobby sitting on the exam table. "Sitting" was really a misnomer as Bobby squirmed constantly and couldn't track well with Dr. X's questions. At various points, Bobby jumped down from the table to run around the exam room, making the interview difficult. I could tell that Dr. X was strategizing how to proceed.

"Mom, can you tell me why you are here today?" Dr. X asked.

"Bobby's school thinks he has ADHD and wants him medicated," she offered. "I know we've discussed this with you before, but his behavior does seem to be getting worse. He can't sit still in class, and his grades are failing. It's leading to a lot of tension between Bobby and his teacher."

"Well, as you know, Mom, we do things a little differently here, at least as our first go around. We try to make medication the last resort," Dr. X replied.

"I'm not thrilled with the idea of medication either," Bobby's mom replied. "What do you suggest?"

At this point, Dr. X directed her attention to Bobby, who was squirming on the floor. "Bobby, tell me about your favorite foods."

"I love ice cream, chocolate chip cookies, and Frosted Flakes!" Bobby offered enthusiastically, typical for a kid his age. Dr. X turned her head to me and gave me a knowing smile.

"Mom, can you please tell me about Bobby's diet? What do you see him eat?" Dr. X asked.

"Bobby does seem to be a sugar addict, that's for sure. He's become somewhat of a picky eater and really doesn't eat much protein anymore, and never vegetables. But he does love fruit," mom replied.

Dr. X performed as much of a physical exam on a wiggling Bobby as she could. She then stood up from the exam stool and indicated that she and I would come back into the room soon. She motioned for me to follow her out the door. I gave Bobby's mom a little wave as I shut the door behind me.

Once back in her office and out of the earshot of Bobby and his mother, Dr. X began to impart her unorthodox approach to ADHD. "Liz, I can't tell you how many of these kids I see in my practice. It's approaching an epidemic. Medications can be dicey, and I am not personally convinced that they should be used in children. My husband and I have developed our own unique approach to this diagnosis, with impressive results. The only drawback? The kids really don't like it," she finished.

Dr. X grabbed a packet of papers from a metal filing cabinet in her office, and we headed back into Bobby's exam room. Once there, she began to explain her desired plan for Bobby's care. "Mom, we've known each other for ten years. You know we don't like to medicate children in this practice. Dr. Y and I have developed a new program for children such as Bobby, and I'd like to share it with you."

As Bobby continued to loudly run around the exam room, Dr. X gave him a couple of tongue blades to play with while she addressed his mother. Bobby sat down on the floor and immediately started to break the tongue blades into pieces.

"Mom, we have had great success treating ADHD with diet alone. Dr. Y and I have a program for Bobby that should help manage his behavior," Dr. X said as she handed the packet of papers to her.

"Diet? What kind of diet?" Bobby's mom asked. "He doesn't need to lose weight, that's for sure. I'm confused."

"Well, the easiest answer is 'no sugar,' and very low carbohydrate," Dr X replied. A keto-type diet was relatively unusual at that time, and rarely, if ever, recommended for a child. "I know it may sound crazy, but a change in Bobby's diet could make a *real* difference for him and you," she stated.

This conversation about diet caught Bobby's attention. He looked up from the broken tongue blades on the floor and responded by shouting at his mom, "No! I won't do it! You can't make me!"

Dr. X gave Bobby a new supply of tongue blades before turning her attention back to Bobby's mother. She then took the packet of information back from her and reviewed it with her in detail. Page after page of "eat this, don't eat that." The handouts also included the names of a couple of keto cookbooks and a referral to an enlightened, like-minded nutritionist.

"To be honest, this diet will be most difficult for you, Mom," Dr. X confessed. "It's hard to deny your child the foods he loves the most, but it really is essential for his healing. I'd like to see you and Bobby weekly for a few visits to see how he is doing on his new program."

"I'll certainly *try* this new diet," Bobby's mother said with a sigh as she took the paperwork from Dr. X.

We exited the room together, and Dr. X gave Bobby's mom a friendly hug goodbye and said, "Good luck! And keep the faith!" I was impressed with how she had handled the whole visit.

Over the next week, I took it upon myself to learn more about ADHD. People with a diagnosis of ADHD exhibit differences in brain function in areas regulating attention, impulse control, and executive functioning. The diagnosis is made by clinical assessments, input from the parents and teachers (most commonly), and meeting the Diagnostic and Statistical Manual (DSM) criteria. To be diagnosed with ADHD, the child must show symptoms in multiple settings, such as school *and* home, and must be diagnosed before age 12. Interestingly, many children with ADHD have higher-than-average IQs.

Bobby exhibited all three potential types of ADHD behaviors: inattention, impulsivity, and hyperactivity, making his symptoms somewhat more challenging to manage and treat. I also learned that ADHD may be exaggerated by certain social situations, like a school classroom, or anywhere a child would be subject to rules and expectations. Children with ADHD exhibiting these behaviors are not volitional, and they benefit from positive reinforcement, structured routines, and clear expectations. Dr. X imparted the wisdom that a change in his diet could also positively affect Bobby's symptoms and behavior.

A week later, we saw Bobby again. The tension in the exam room was obvious as we entered. Bobby was sitting and squirming on the floor. His mom was sitting on a chair and looked exhausted and somewhat defeated.

"Mom, how did last week go for Bobby?" Dr. X asked, already intuiting the answer from an obviously frustrated mother.

"Horrible! I hate the food!" Bobby interjected and exclaimed. "I want M&Ms!" Bobby then asked Dr. X, "Can I have more of those sticks?"

Dr. X grabbed a few tongue blades from the cabinet and handed them to Bobby. "Here you go, sweetie. I'm going to talk to your mom now."

"Honestly, Dr. X, it was a really difficult week," Mom confessed. "We did our best. His behavior has been a *tiny* bit better, but the constant fighting over food and meals 24/7 has been exhausting, to say the least."

"All of this is expected," Dr. X offered. "Sugar is one of the most addictive substances a human can eat, and getting off of it can be extremely difficult, especially for a child. Hold the faith, Mom, and keep Bobby on the diet. We will see you again in a week."

Dr. X continued to educate me once we left the exam room. She shared how she and her husband had had to put their own son on the keto diet for ADHD, which was the genesis of their unconventional program. "Liz, I've lived this, that which I am asking Bobby and his mother to do. It sucks. Big time. But our program really *can* work if the patient and their family are very committed. My main goal for these past two weeks has really just been to get them to recognize how much sugar he was really consuming. It's an education that takes time, and it has to be lived."

A week later, we saw Bobby again. This time, when we entered the room, Bobby was sitting quietly on the exam table, playing with a small toy.

"Hi Bobby! Hi Mom, how was last week?" Dr. X asked as she sat down on the exam stool.

"To be honest, it was the best week we have had in a long time. Bobby's teacher even sent me an email and commented on his improved behavior in class," Mom offered. "She actually assumed we had put Bobby on medication."

"How is the diet going?" Dr. X asked, knowing it would take a couple of weeks for Bobby to enter any semblance of "ketosis," the ultimate goal of the diet.

"Much better. Bobby isn't fighting the diet so much anymore and is trying to follow your instructions. And I actually think *he* feels better," Mom replied. "The hardest part is school lunches. He hates that I make him eat a packed lunch. I do think he 'cheats' a bit at school. He even confessed to me that he traded his cheese stick for a peanut butter cup the other day."

"First of all, Mom, great job. I can see a noticeable improvement in Bobby's behavior in just the past couple of weeks. Our goal is to minimize cheating, but we know it's a tough diet for a kid to follow. If he can stay on the diet, you should expect to see sustained and continued improvement in his behavior. For Bobby and his young brain, sugar is poison," Dr. X finished. This forthright comment elicited a nod of agreement from Bobby's mom.

I was able to see Bobby for a total of four visits while on this family practice rotation. His reduction of ADHD symptoms correlated with his adherence to the no sugar, ketogenic diet. I was impressed with the unorthodox approach to a too common affliction, and with Bobby's rapidly improving symptoms. As I continued my tenure as a medical student, I didn't see another medical practitioner recommend diet modification for ADHD, and it certainly wasn't taught in medical school.

Nutrition education in medical schools is widely acknowledged as insufficient, despite the critical role diet plays in preventing and managing chronic diseases. In 1985, a minimum of 25 hours over four years in nutrition education was recommended for medical students. But most U.S. schools have consistently fallen short, with some schools offering little education in nutrition at all.

And, the trend has worsened over time. A 2023 survey found that 58% of medical students received *no* nutrition education whatsoever. This gap leaves physicians underprepared to counsel patients on diet, with only 14% of all doctors feeling comfortable discussing nutrition with their patients.

The more I learned about nutrition by self-study, the more I appreciated and respected Drs. X & Y for their knowledge, courage, and unusual care of their patients.

Chapter 4
A Very Bad Diagnosis

When I interviewed for medical school, one of my meetings was with the Chief of Head & Neck Surgery at the university, an irreverent and boisterous man. I must have done well in the interview, despite Dr. Surgery's oddball questions, because I was admitted to the school on my first attempt. I didn't see my interviewer for several years after our pre-admission meeting, as he performed only the most challenging head and neck cases at the institution. He rarely lets medical students into his operating room. He was an intimidating man, and most of us students seldom saw him.

One day, in my third year of medical school, while on a hospital clinical rotation, I ran into Dr. Surgery walking the halls of the hospital. He said hello and stopped to have a conversation with me.

"Hi Liz, how is school going for you?" he asked sincerely. "I heard you are near the top of your class. Is that true?"

I was impressed that he remembered me, and more impressed that he was aware of my class standing. I wasn't sure where he was heading with his line of questioning. We had just received our class rankings from our first two years of medical school, and I was reported to be in the top 10% of the class, something that must have impressed him.

"Yes, that's what I heard, too, Dr. Surgery," I replied, feeling both proud of the accomplishment and embarrassed in front of him.

"Well, I have a *really* big case coming up tomorrow. Would you like to join me in the operating room?" he asked. I couldn't believe he was actually inviting me to join him in the OR, a goal I had had since the day he interviewed me.

I was surprised and delighted at the invitation. Dr. Surgery's reputation preceded him, and he was known as the maverick who would take on cases that all other surgeons had passed on. Dr. Surgery was talented and skilled, for sure, but it was his confidence and arrogance that buoyed him to perform these high-risk procedures that no one else would touch. I assumed his "big case" was one such patient, and I was excited at being asked to join him.

"That would be great!" I replied.

"Good, meet me tomorrow in the operating suite at the VA at 6 a.m. sharp. Be sure to put something in your stomach and use the bathroom before you scrub in, it's going to be a very long case," he finished. We parted ways in the hallway and went about our day. I realized that I had forgotten to ask him *what* surgery he had planned, so there was little I could do to study or prepare ahead of time. I assumed there would be teaching during the case, as there usually is.

The next day, I arrived at the hospital at 5 a.m., wanting to ensure that I wouldn't be late for the surgery. I put on hospital scrubs and headed to the operating suite of the VA. I ran into Dr. Surgery at the large sink area where you scrub in before entering the sterile OR.

"Hey Liz, so glad that you could make it today. We have a challenging case of advanced throat cancer in a 65-year-old man. Are you ready to watch my magic?" he asked with a confident grin as he vigorously scrubbed his hands and lower arms with the iodine.

"I think so," I replied cheerily. *Hmmm. Throat cancer. That's a diagnosis I hadn't seen before or prepared for,* I thought as I cleaned my own skin. I wondered what this maverick had planned for his patient, obviously hoping to give him a chance to live a longer life when all other doctors had likely given up on him.

Dr. Surgery and I stood side by side at the sink and scrubbed our hands and arms with the provided soap and iodine before entering the operating suite. Once inside, I noticed the patient on the table, already anesthetized and waiting for Dr. Surgery. In addition to the anesthesiologist, the table was surrounded by two other doctors, in various years of residency training, who were attending to the patient while waiting for the chief to arrive. With the help of a scrub nurse, Dr. Surgery and I put on our sterile gown, hat, and gloves, and approached the table.

"Hi everyone, we have a visitor with us today, Liz. She is a medical student and will be assisting me. Can we please get her a stool to stand on?" he asked the head scrub nurse. A stool appeared out of nowhere and was placed at the head of the table opposite where Dr. Surgery would be working. Before the first cut was made, he had more requests of the team. "Please put on my music, and place the patient's MRI scan results in the lightbox." A scrub nurse placed a CD in a CD player in the OR and pushed "play." Most surgeons like to have their favorite music played in the background while they operate. Van Halen, Mozart, Billy Joel, etc.

The surgeon's musical preference took precedence in the OR, and all of the others there would get to "enjoy" the music throughout the case, whether they liked the music or not. At times, the surgeon will ask for silence as he or she works during a particularly delicate or difficult part of the operation. During those times, you can hear a pin drop in the room.

The head surgeon is in charge of the operating room, and there is a strict hierarchy to be followed, similar to a Captain of an airplane. As a medical student, you are instructed to be seen, but not heard. You do what you are told, you keep your mouth shut, and only speak when spoken to. And, you should never ask questions of the chief during the actual surgery. All that, in addition to learning how to hold a tissue retractor for hours on end, was the only way to survive time in the OR.

As a medical student, you are truly at the bottom of the totem pole. If you are addressed by the chief, it is usually to be "pimped" to see how much you know about anatomy and any particular disease. If you break the rules of OR decorum, you could be banished from the procedure, get yelled at in front of the team, or even have a retractor or other medical instrument thrown your way. At this time in the early to mid-1990s, the OR was still very much a "man's world," and the testosterone levels were always high.

I took my place on the stool at the head of the bed across from Dr. Surgery. As we gazed down at the patient's head below us, we could see the right side of his face and neck peeking out of the sterile drapes. Dr. Surgery handed me a scalpel, and I froze. *You want me to make the first cut? Are you for real?* I thought to myself and began to panic.

"Just kidding, Lizzy," he replied jokingly as he took the scalpel back from me and rolled his eyes. "You are in charge of the retractor, a *very* important job."

Whew, thank God for that! I said to myself as I remained quiet.

"This case is going to be long, Liz. This man has stage 4 carcinoma of his trachea and windpipe. The cancer was also found on his vocal cords. I am the fourth surgeon he has seen in consultation, and the only one willing to try and help him surgically. After we remove the cancer, we are going to have to fashion him a new throat using part of his intestines. It's his only chance of survival at this point, as chemotherapy and radiation have not helped, and no one else is willing to operate on him," he finished.

Ah, there's the teaching I was waiting for, admitting to myself that the information imparted really didn't help me with understanding the complex procedure. I kept quiet and waited for the surgical ballet to begin.

Dr. Surgery took the scalpel and began to cut the patient's tissue from his right ear down to his right clavicle. From there, and with the help of my stellar retractor holding, he carefully and meticulously dissected his entire neck. It reminded me of the cadaver lab, only this patient was still alive, and blood replaced formaldehyde. The dissection took hours to accurately locate the cancer, and once found, Dr. Surgery carefully removed the diseased tissue bit by bit. The cancer itself was chalky white and very friable, making it easy to identify.

Stage 4 throat cancer is a really bad diagnosis. Tumor spread and lymph node involvement impart a worse outcome, as was the case with this patient. Throat cancer can present in a variety of ways, with a sore throat, difficulty swallowing, and hoarseness as common symptoms. In advanced cases, ear pain, difficulty breathing, and weight loss can be seen. The most common cause, as it was for our patient, is a history of heavy smoking and concomitant alcohol consumption. Additionally, the human papillomavirus is almost always found in mouth and throat cancers.

With stage 4 cancer of the throat, our patient's five-year survival rate was around 30%, and the likelihood of recurrence was around 50%. It is one of the most devastating diagnoses due to the poor prognosis and extensive disfigurement that comes with surgery. This type of cancer can also make eating difficult, and these patients usually require supplemental nutrition through a tube placed directly into their stomach.

After several hours of holding the tissue retractor, Dr. Surgeon indicated he was nearly finished with his extensive dissection. By this point, it had become clear to me what all of the other people surrounding the table were up to. Dr.

Surgery let me know that the general surgery team was performing a simultaneous operation on the patient's abdomen, retrieving the small bowel tissue he would need to reconstruct the patient's windpipe.

"How are you guys doing down there?" Dr. Surgeon asked the team at the patient's abdomen.

"Pretty good, sir, we are almost done with the resection," a senior resident surgeon answered.

Thank God for that, I thought to myself. We were already five hours into the procedure, and I had to pee. I reminded myself to skip the coffee the next time I'm scrubbed into the operating room.

Rock music blared from the CD player, and Dr. Surgeon began to wiggle his legs to the rhythm as we waited. One of the hardest parts of surgery is the prolonged standing in one place that is required, sometimes exceeding ten hours or more. My legs were aching, so I began to wiggle too.

"Are we having fun yet, Liz?" Dr. Surgery asked with a smile. "I warned you this was going to be a long case."

"I am fine, sir," I replied, understanding that was the only acceptable answer I could provide. Medical students are not allowed to complain in the OR, or pretty much anywhere else. Quiet compliance is expected.

"James, are you ready to hand me that small bowel yet?" Dr. Surgery asked impatiently of the resident surgeon located at the patient's abdomen.

"Yes, sir, here it is," James replied as he handed Dr. Surgery a five-inch length of bowel that looked like tripe.

Dr. Surgery took the piece of colon and spread it out on an adjacent sterile table to examine and clean the bowel carefully. In this experimental procedure, the patient will end up with part of their colon in their throat. This leads to a host of other problems, like constant mucus and phlegm, but it was his only shot at life. As the cancer had spread to his vocal cords, he would eventually need another surgery to address that issue with a "voice box." But, for today, our only goal was to remove the cancer completely and place the piece of colon in his throat.

By the ninth hour, standing over the patient holding the retractor, I was hungry and exhausted. As we were finishing up the case, Dr. Surgeon stopped his sewing and handed me the suture and suggested that I complete the case. I had watched Dr. Surgeon's suturing technique closely, and did my best to emulate him for the few sutures he let me place.

"Hey, you sew pretty good… for a girl!" Dr. Surgeon exclaimed loudly to the room as I finished the last suture.

Was that hazing? Overt sexism? Not knowing how to respond, I kept quiet. Soon thereafter, we were allowed to remove our sterile garb and exit the OR after a ten-hour operation. I nearly ran to the bathroom, and my legs felt like jelly.

After the extensive surgery, I still had to see my own list of patients in the hospital, making for an exceptionally long, 16-hour day. I arrived home at 9 p.m. and fell into bed without eating dinner. My husband asked me about my day, but I found it difficult to explain to him what I had just witnessed - and participated in. How do I explain this to a non-medical person? I had to admit to myself that the surgery was gruesome, disfiguring, and this patient's only chance at life. Words escaped me. How do you tactfully describe a prolonged and poignant surgery to someone not in the medical profession? I fell asleep before I came up with the answer.

The next day, I arrived at the hospital at 6 a.m. to see my own patients. As I was compiling my patient list for the day, I received a page from Dr. Surgeon. It said, "Call me, Liz."

I dutifully called Dr. Surgeon back, surprised to hear from him.

"Liz, thank you for joining me yesterday in the OR, I appreciate your help with the retractor. I know you are not assigned to this patient, but I wanted you to know that he did not survive the night," he reported.

"Oh, wow, that sucks," I replied. Even though I had never met the patient while he was awake, after 10 hours with him in the OR, I had become attached to his hopefully positive outcome.

"Yep. You win some, you lose some, Liz," he replied with resignation and without emotion. "Have a great day," he said before hanging up the phone. A response perfectly in keeping with his maverick reputation. It took me a little longer to process the bad outcome.

That was the first and only time I was able to join Dr. Surgery in the operating room.

Chapter 5
A Terrible Aim

Training to be a medical doctor is rigorous. Intentionally so. Little sleep, infrequent meals, and an avalanche of information to grasp and retain. The information comes at you so fast, and you have to assimilate that knowledge as soon as possible.

The depth and breadth of what you are expected to learn – and be competent at - is frequently overwhelming, but an accepted part of being a doctor in training. There's an adage in medicine: "See one, do one, teach one." Meaning, you are expected to learn a procedure by watching it, perform said procedure on your own, and then teach it to another learner. Medicine doesn't suffer fools or slow learners.

An area often overlooked or long-forgotten by the higher-ups in medicine (aka the "attending physician") is the emotional roller coaster you ride in medical training. Bad outcomes despite best efforts can really weigh on you, especially early in your training, before you have "toughened up." My next patient, Mr. Lee, was one such patient who took me on such a ride.

I was in my third year of medical school, assigned to the university's plastic surgery department. It was still relatively early in my training, and I had visited very few patients myself in the hospital at that point. My boss - Dr. Repair - was a plastic surgeon who specialized in facial and body reconstruction after traumatic accidents, or disfiguring diagnoses such as cancer. He prided himself on restoring his patients' appearance to their pre-trauma, or pre-disease state, as much as possible. And, he was reportedly very, very good at it.

Dr. Repair was a perfectionist who demanded perfection from his residents and students on his service. As the facility was a teaching hospital, we were thrown in with the mix of patients who were going to have facial and/or body reconstructive plastic surgery, not aesthetic plastic surgery.

As a medical student, spending time with Dr. Repair in the operating room was a reward for hard and accurate work on the wards. If Dr. Repair felt you deserved time with him in the OR, he would invite you to join him. If he didn't, you were left out and relegated full-time to the pre- and post-op care of the patients on the wards, either waiting for, or recovering from, the plastic surgical procedure.

One early morning, about six a.m., while pre-rounding on my patients, Dr. Repair approached me where I was sitting at the nurse's station and said, "Hey, do you want to join me today in the OR?"

As this was a coveted activity on this rotation, I quickly said, "Absolutely!"

Dr. Repair informed me that we would be doing a breast reconstruction post-double mastectomy on a 45-year-old breast cancer patient. He told me to "study up" on the procedure before joining him in the OR in an hour. I happily complied and headed to the library to do some research before the surgery.

At the appointed time, I changed into scrubs and began my walk from the resident's room to the suite of operating rooms to meet up with Dr. Repair. I weaved my way to the large sink area where surgeons scrub in before entering the sterile operating suite. Dr. Repair stood next to me at the sink and watched my technique of sterilizing my hands and arms. I watched Dr. Repair's technique and tried to emulate him the best I could, taking extra care to scrub under my fingernails, like him. I scrubbed my hands and arms so vigorously with the provided anti-septic soap and sponge that I thought I might peel off my skin.

As we scrubbed ourselves, Dr. Repair indicated the breast reconstruction case had been bumped by a new patient with an emergency. Not wanting to pry, I didn't ask for any more information about the case, and dutifully followed him into the OR.

Once in the operating room, we donned our sterile gowns, gloves, and masks while waiting for the patient to be brought from the emergency department to the operating suite. At this point, Dr. Repair told me we would be working on a patient who had tried to commit suicide. I was intrigued as to why this patient needed a reconstructive plastic surgeon. It didn't take long before I was hit with the grim reality of what had happened to this patient.

Mr. Lee was a 28-year-old Asian man. He worked in high tech and had recently lost his job and girlfriend. He became so despondent that he had decided the solution was to use a hunting gun to kill himself. He took a shotgun and aimed it under his chin, facing straight up.

When Mr. Lee used the firearm, he managed to blow off his entire face while missing most of his brain, but he didn't die. Literally, his face was gone: no eyes, no nose, and no mouth. All I could see were holes where those features used to be, and some exposed brain tissue. He had been intubated in the ER, and it was a gruesome miracle that he was still alive. Now it was Dr. Repair's job to keep him alive.

I don't remember much from that operation as I processed the trauma I was witnessing. I dutifully held the retractor as Dr. Repair took nine hours to carefully reconstruct Mr. Lee's tissue to give him a fighting chance at life. Skin grafts from other parts of his body were employed to stem the damage and cover the exposed brain tissue as much as possible. The surgery was a "success" in that the patient survived the surgery. I left the OR exhausted from standing in place for nine hours, and quickly looked for a bathroom before foraging for food.

As I was the primary medical student assisting Dr. Repair in the OR, Mr. Lee became "my patient" for the duration of my month-long rotation in plastic surgery. Meaning, it was my responsibility to see him daily and report his progress - or decline - to Dr. Repair.

I saw Mr. Lee every day, and we began conversations after a week or so. Communicating with him was extremely difficult as half of his tongue had been vaporized, and he had lost the front half of his teeth as well, so we were left to communicate by pen and paper. It was surreal to interact with someone who had no facial features save five holes in his face: two eye sockets, two holes where his nose used to be, and a large hole where his mouth once was. His face resembled a patchwork quilt of new tissue from the attempts to reform his facial features. He had a feeding tube placed directly into his stomach as he was unable to eat.

Mr. Lee's appearance was jarring and disconcerting at first, but as usual in medicine, you become somewhat hardened and "used to" the state of your patients. Over time, I spoke with Mr. Lee a lot about the suicide attempt. He was extremely angry and depressed that his attempt had failed, and now he was still alive without a face. He was furious with himself for not knowing how to point the gun. He wrote of death and dying each time I met with him, and he refused any pharmacologic or psychological interventions for his depression.

Suicide and suicide attempts are a serious concern for doctors and society at large. Depression, anxiety, and substance use are the primary drivers of this phenomenon, with 13 million Americans contemplating suicide each year, 1.5 million attempting suicide, and 50 thousand fatalities occurring each year. This amounts to about one death by suicide every 11 minutes in the U.S.

Men make up 79% of all suicides and use guns primarily for their act. Men are four times more likely than women to die from a suicide attempt due to the use of guns, which have a 90% fatality rate. Women most commonly attempt suicide by an overdose of pills, with a death rate of 13%. When it comes to suicide, men are far more "successful" than women due to the weapon of choice. Firearms are usually fatal.

The cause of suicide is multifactorial, encompassing economic, social, psychological, and environmental influences. An inverted bell curve sheds more light on the problem, with the youngest and oldest in today's society most vulnerable to suicide. Suicide rates are highest in whites and American Indians, and the lowest rates are seen in blacks and Asians. Mr. Lee was an unusual suicide patient as he was both Asian and unsuccessful in using a gun in his suicide attempt.

At the time of meeting Mr. Lee, a national suicide hotline did not exist. Since that time, there has been a major national effort to streamline a response to this epidemic. The advent of the "988 Suicide and Crisis Lifeline" has been a positive step forward in providing support and services to those contemplating suicide.

When I rotated off the plastic surgery service a month after Mr. Lee's first operation, he had started to come out of his shell. I would occasionally see him walking the halls of the ward, completely face-free. He was completely blind and needed assistance with walking. The team on the ward - and other patients - had become used to seeing his unusual and grotesquely-formed appearance.

On my final day of my rotation in plastic surgery, I spent a bit more time with Mr. Lee, saddened that I wouldn't be able to round on him anymore. I wondered who would pick up with him where I was leaving off. Mr. Lee, now having had repeated surgeries to reform any semblance of a face, told me he couldn't wait to be discharged, so that he could "finish the job" he had started a month earlier.

Given his present state, I really couldn't argue with his plan, but I kept my feelings to myself.

Chapter 6
Medical Sleuth

Sometimes being a medical student is a good thing. As a student, you have a support structure above you to hopefully guide your learning and lend assistance when needed. Generally, you are given fewer patients to care for than your more learned and senior colleagues. This extra time with your patient grants you access to more time interviewing your patient. Sometimes, this extra time means that you just might be the detective who "solves the case," as was the situation with my next patient.

I was in the middle of my third year of medical school and was finishing up my required clinical rotations for the year. I felt fortunate by that time in my training that I had seen an incredible variety of maladies and illnesses that helped me feel somewhat competent at managing so many different diagnoses.

My inpatient general pediatric rotation was next, and I approached this rotation with unusual confidence. I was starting to feel comfortable with the common diagnoses that require hospitalization. I was also excited to work with Dr. Jones, the pediatric attending. He had a reputation for being a good teacher and kind to his team of learners.

All of that confidence and excitement disappeared one morning at 7 a.m., when my attending assigned me to a new admission. "Liz, I'd like you to admit our next patient. His name is Andrew and he is 13 years old. He is in the emergency department and will be in room #414 soon. He is having trouble breathing, and the X-ray in the ED does not look good. Please see him and come find me with your proposed workup before you write your admission note and orders."

I went to the nearest computer and pulled up Andrew's X-ray. Something major was certainly going on, but it didn't look like a typical, garden-variety, community-acquired pneumonia. He also had an elevated white count and a high fever of 102 degrees. I called the emergency department and asked for his estimated time of arrival to the wards. The ED secretary let me know that Andrew was already on his way up to the pediatric floor.

While still sitting at the nurse's station, Andrew was wheeled past me on a stretcher with his parents in tow. He had an oxygen mask on his face and appeared to be having trouble breathing. I waited for a few minutes for him to be settled in his room, then entered with a quiet knock on the door.

"Hello, my name is Liz, I am a student doctor, here to get you settled in for Dr. Jones," I stated as I held out my hands to greet both parents.

"Hi Liz, can you help us?" Andrew's mother immediately asked in earnest, with a terrified look on her face.

"Yes, I am here to help," I replied. "My team and I will do our absolute best to help your son."

Andrew appeared too uncomfortable to withstand an interview, and it was difficult to understand him through the oxygen mask that he couldn't take off due to his low oxygen saturation. His parents answered most of the questions I asked, and the confirmatory information from Andrew came from nods of his head as his parents spoke.

I learned that Andrew was a normally healthy, typical 13-year-old. He played sports in school, got reasonably good grades, and was known as a popular kid in eighth grade. He had two older siblings living at home who were healthy. Andrew's illness had come on quickly in the days before admission to the hospital. He came home from football practice with a fever and body aches about a week before this admission.

Andrew's parents assumed he had a "normal" illness, such as a cold or flu, and kept him home from school for a couple of days. His symptoms worsened, and a new, non-productive cough and headaches commenced. Tylenol and Ibuprofen didn't break the fever, so they took him to urgent care. There, he was given a cough suppressant, a mild antibiotic, and was sent home.

Once home, Andrew's condition continued to worsen, and he began to have difficulty breathing. His fever reached 103 degrees. His parents called his primary pediatrician, who had recommended they take Andrew to the ER. Now here, admitted to the hospital, it was my job to put together what was going on. I spent most of my time talking with the parents, trying to rule out or rule in a definitive diagnosis.

Andrew appeared to live a normal, uneventful 13-year-old life. In front of his parents, Andrew denied any illicit drug or alcohol use by shaking his head "no" to questions when I asked him directly. I completed a physical exam on Andrew and made a note of his low oxygen saturation despite being on supplemental oxygen at four litres per minute. Something bad was certainly going on.

After my interview and physical exam, I tucked Andrew in for the moment and looked for my attending. I found him at the nurse's station, working on the computer. "Hi, Dr. Jones, I am finished with Andrew. Is now a good time to discuss him?" I asked.

"Sure, Liz, I've got a couple of minutes. What's going on with him?" he asked.

"Well, all signs point to a community-acquired pneumonia. But, it appears urgent care prescribed him an ineffective antibiotic four days ago," I replied. "It looks to me like he needs a broad-spectrum IV antibiotic, and possibly steroids. His X-ray is abnormal and unusual, and it really doesn't look like a typical pneumonia," I finished.

"I agree. The chest X-ray is indeed concerning. The antibiotic sounds good, but let's hold off on the steroid. Let's also get a spiral CT scan of his chest," he said. I thanked him for his time and went back to Andrew's room to discuss the plan with his family and him. I also started him on two "big gun" antibiotics that should have covered most any bacterial pathogen.

I continued to follow Andrew for a couple of days, but to my surprise, he didn't improve at all, and he continued to have a high fever and low oxygen saturation. His case was vexing to my attending, as well. Each morning during rounds, we discussed what could be causing his illness. We even discussed amongst ourselves the idea that Andrew may need to be intubated and put on a ventilator if he didn't improve. This possibility terrified his parents.

After rounds one day, I decided that I better do a little more detective work to see if there was any stone left unturned. Something I had missed that would unlock the mystery of Andrew's illness. I returned to his room and was pleased to see that we were alone. His parents had stepped away to get coffee from the cafeteria. This would be our first time speaking privately.

"Hi, Andrew," I said as I entered the room. He was sitting up in bed with his oxygen mask on. His breathing was labored, and he looked concerned. "I'm glad we have some time alone," I stated.

Andrew gave me a little wave as I sat down next to him. "Andrew, I need to ask you some questions again that I asked you when your parents were here," I continued. "I need you to be completely honest with me."

"Okay, what do you want to know?" he asked through labored breaths behind the mask.

"Do you use *any* drugs?" I implored, staring directly at him. "I promise you; you will not get in trouble for telling me the truth. But the truth may help us in your care."

Andrew turned his head away from me and said through the mask, "Yes, I smoke pot, but my parents don't know. They would *kill* me if they knew."

"Thank you for your honesty, Andrew. *How* do you smoke pot?" I replied.

"I have a bong hidden in my room. Our house is pretty big, so no one knows when I do it," he offered. "I pretty much use it every day."

"*Where* do you hide your bong, Andrew?" I asked. I was beginning to feel hopeful for the first time about Andrew's malady.

"It's in my closet, in a shoe box," he replied.

"Thank you for sharing this information with me. I am going to ask your parents to bring in the bong for testing," I finished. I had had no personal experience with illicit drugs up to that point in my life, but I hoped his apparatus would help unravel the mystery pneumonia.

I met up with Andrew's parents in the hallway and had the difficult conversation with them about the marijuana. They were unsurprisingly upset, but glad to know. They agreed to go home to locate and bring in the bong.

Next, I paged Dr. Jones to update him on my medical sleuthing. I was excited to share with him my idea about the bong. I found him in the hospital's cafeteria. "Hi, Dr. Jones. I think I may have found the culprit in Andrew's case," I shared as I sat down at his table. "He smokes pot regularly and uses a bong. I have asked his parents to bring the bong into the hospital for pathogen testing."

"That might be the stupidest thing I have ever heard from a medical student. I expected more from you, Liz," he admonished between bites of food. "Did you miss mycoplasma? The last thing we need in this hospital is a bong." He turned his attention back to a newspaper he was reading, indicating our conversation was over.

I was crestfallen and felt the wind leave my intellectual sails. *Of course*, I had thought about Mycoplasma pneumonia and had covered Andrew with the appropriate antibiotic for that bug, a fact that my attending should have known. My thinking was *beyond* a bacterial infection, as Andrew had not improved on the antibiotic for mycoplasma.

I tried not to take the harsh words from my supervisor too personally. Just a few short years before, such feedback would have brought tears to my eyes. But now, hardened by three years of grueling schoolwork and education, I simply turned on my heels and swallowed my pride, at least temporarily.

The next day, Andrew's parents brought me a bath towel-wrapped glass bong. The inside of the glass was covered in a smelly, black goo that was sticky when touched. It appeared that Andrew may not have *ever* cleaned the bong, a fact he later confirmed for me. He also told me that he bought his pot through various friends at school, many of whom grew their own marijuana.

I took Andrew's bong myself to the lab in the hospital. I met with the lab manager and told her of my diagnostic dilemma. She let me know that all kinds of mold and fungi can grow on surfaces where marijuana has been smoked. She said it was likely that "something bad" was growing within the molded glass. She asked me to leave the bong with her, so I did.

The tests in the lab were fruitful and ultimately allowed us to make a definitive diagnosis for Andrew. His recreational activity, using a dirty bong to repeatedly smoke illicit marijuana, had given him a terrible case of pulmonary *Aspergillus*. This is a fungus commonly found in homegrown marijuana, the only type of marijuana available at that time. When the fungus cultures came back, we were able to stop his antibiotics and put him on the appropriate antifungal. Andrew's condition improved quickly after the medication adjustment, and after a few more days, he was finally able to be discharged home.

One day, towards the end of my rotation, Dr. Jones approached me before our 7 a.m. morning meeting and spoke to me privately. "Hey Liz, I've been meaning to tell you, good work on the bong case," he said. "I was wrong to criticize you, and your crazy sleuthing allowed us to actually help Andrew. Good job."

It is times like that, and words like those, that make it all worthwhile: the sleepless nights, the time away from family and friends, the hazing, and the exhaustion. Actually, helping a patient get better trumps all that.

"Thank you very much, Dr. Jones. Your words mean a lot," I replied as we entered the room together for our daily meeting.

Chapter 7
Anything, But This

In my third year of medical school, and before I gave birth to my first child, I was assigned to an outpatient neurology rotation.

The neurologist, Dr. Brain, had recently arrived in town from the East Coast, and I was excited to work with him. His name and copious credentials were legendary in textbooks and journal articles. But it was his personality that I was excited to experience. Dr. Brain had the reputation of being exceptionally kind, other-worldly, smart, and easy to work with. I looked forward to a good month.

On my first day of the rotation, I arrived early at Dr. Brain's office. I entered the waiting room and was struck by the beautiful furnishings, the original artwork, and the incredible wall fountain. I knew by that point in my training that most visits to a neurologist are rarely good, with innumerable devastating diagnoses at play. I wondered if the opulence and beauty of the waiting room were in an attempt to offset the delivery of bad news to the patient who would eventually sit there.

The waiting room was empty, and the receptionist greeted me with a welcoming smile. "Hi! You must be Liz," she said as I approached the desk in my self-identifying short, white coat. "I'm Susan."

"Hi Susan, yes, that's me," I replied with a smile. "Nice to meet you."

"Dr. Brain is waiting for you in his office. Head through this door and you will find him at the end of the hall in the corner office," she finished.

I found Dr. Brain in his office dictating a chart note from a recent patient. He looked up at me and gave me a big smile before rising to greet me. "You must be Liz," he stated as he shook my hand enthusiastically. "So glad you are here. We have a busy month ahead," he continued. "Have a seat, and we will prepare for the day."

I sat down in a chair directly facing Dr. Brain, who was sitting behind his desk. He appeared to be a well-preserved man in his 60s and was quite handsome. He let me know he had moved to the West Coast to follow his now wife, giving up a prestigious post at an Ivy League university to marry her. He asked me about my life, and obvious pregnancy, and gave me his enthusiastic support for starting a family. I appreciated his words more than he knew.

Dr. Brain then started to tell me the skinny on a neurology practice. The specialty sees some of the most devastating diagnoses in all of medicine. Neurology patients' diagnoses are often chronic, life-long afflictions with very few good treatments at that time, and even fewer cures. He told me that I would be seeing a wide variety of neurological illnesses and diseases. We then reviewed the patient census for the day and discussed individual illnesses, if known. My head was swimming from all of the diseases and diagnoses I had yet to learn.

At that point, Dr. Brain's nurse came to his door and let him know his first patient was waiting in exam room #3. "Thank you, Carol, we will be right in," he stated.

"Liz, I'd like you to go see this patient by yourself first while I finish up my dictation," Dr. Brain stated. "He is a new patient to our clinic, so I'd like you to see if you can figure out what is going on with him."

I wasn't sure if I should be flattered or terrified on my first day of the rotation. "No problem, Dr. Brain, I'll go see him now," I replied, feeling completely inept and unprepared for meeting the new patient alone.

I knocked on the door of exam room #3 and opened it slowly. I was expecting to see a single patient, but a very handsome, obviously well-to-do, middle-aged couple greeted me instead. "Hi, I'm Liz, a student doctor working with Dr. Brain. He has asked me to speak with you first," I stated. Oftentimes, the addition of a medical student thrown into the mix is met with resistance by the patient, but this time, I was welcomed.

"Please tell me what brings you in today to see Dr. Brain," I asked. Rarely, if a patient was in a bad mood or was cynical, I might hear "a car" in response to that question. This day, the mood was more serious, and they answered my question without sarcasm.

"We are here because my husband has been having problems," his wife answered. I realized at that point that I should direct my questions to the patient specifically, only relying on his wife for corroborating information.

The patient was a 55-year-old man named Bruce. He was self-employed in the construction business and had built several of the high-rise buildings in our city. He and his wife had been married for 30 years and had four children. They owned a home in Hawaii and traveled extensively for business and pleasure. Bruce drank alcohol occasionally and did not smoke or use drugs. He was very fit for his age and reported working out daily in his home gym. He denied any hazardous occupational exposures. Overall, his history was unremarkable.

"Bruce, please tell me in your own words what you have been experiencing," I said.

"Well, I've always been 'one of the guys' at work; helping my team with heavy lifting, construction equipment, and more. About a year ago, I started to have weakness in my left arm and both legs. It was barely noticeable at first, but it seems to have gotten worse, and now it's hard to help out my crew due to my weakness," Bruce reported. "I also now have an occasional tremor in my left hand, which is why my primary care doctor sent me here."

"He dropped and broke a wine glass last week due to the tremor," Bruce's wife offered. "He also slurs his words on occasion, even when he hasn't had a sip of wine." His wife had just given me two incredibly important pieces of information that I was sure would mean something major to Dr. Brain.

I delved into Bruce's family history, but it was unremarkable. I then conducted a brief examination of Bruce and performed as much of a neurological exam as I could, with my limited knowledge, experience, and tools. I noted slight weakness of his arms bilaterally, with the left arm weaker than the right arm. His reflexes in his legs were hyperactive, denoting a problem in his nervous system. His Babinski reflexes were positive bilaterally, indicating a significant neurological deficit of some origin.

Once I had completed as much of the physical examination as I could, I excused myself to return to Dr. Brain's office. "Bruce, I'm going to go get Dr. Brain now. He may ask you the same questions, so please think of any other information you might be able to provide to him. You are in great hands, and I'm sure Dr. Brain will be able to get to the bottom of what is causing your symptoms," I finished with as much confidence as I could before exiting the exam room.

I met up with Dr. Brain again in his office. "So, Liz, what do you think is going on with our patient?" he asked me as soon as I sat down.

"To be honest, sir, I'm really not sure," I replied. "He has some neurological signs and symptoms that appear to be getting a bit worse. His biggest deficits are weakness in his legs, a tremor in his left hand, and positive Babinski's sign bilaterally. He's also had some trouble on occasion with slurred speech. I'm not really sure how to put this puzzle together."

"Follow me," Dr. Brain said as he stood up from his desk, threw a stethoscope around his neck, and picked up a traditional "doctor's bag" from his credenza.

We entered Bruce's exam room together. After the requisite introductions, Dr. Brain sat on an exam stool and squarely faced Bruce, who was sitting on the exam table.

"Bruce, Liz has given me a lot of information about your situation. I'm now going to ask you some questions myself," Dr. Brain said.

"Bruce, have you had any other symptoms you can share with me, like muscle twitching, muscle stiffness, or any difficulty breathing?" Dr. Brain asked gently.

"Yes, I do have occasional muscle spasms in my left upper arm, the same side as the problem I had with the wine glass," Bruce replied. "All of my problems seem to have started over the last year."

Dr. Brain then conducted the most thorough physical examination on Bruce that I had yet to witness in medicine. He used various instruments to elicit neurological responses from all parts of his body that seemed to hold great meaning for him. With each new physical exam test, I felt I was witnessing the unfolding of a medical diagnosis by someone much more learned than I. It was humbling to witness the volume of information he was collecting from just a physical exam. I had no idea what Dr. Brain was thinking, and I felt pretty clueless and useless at that point.

"Bruce, Liz and I are going to leave for a few minutes, and then we will be back to share our plan of care with you," Dr. Brain stated.

Dr. Brain and I reconvened in his office. "Well, Liz, any better idea of what is going on with Bruce?" he asked.

"I hate to say it, but I have a gut feeling it's something *really* bad," I replied. "I'm thinking possibly of multiple sclerosis?"

"Not out of the question, but I'm thinking about a different diagnosis: amyotrophic lateral sclerosis (ALS)," he stated.

ALS? Oh wow, I hadn't even thought about that diagnosis and have never seen it before! I thought to myself.

Dr. Brain then proceeded to enlighten me on his working diagnosis. What I learned left me horrified: a devastating diagnosis with a terrible prognosis, delivered to Bruce in the prime of his life. "Let's go speak with them again," he said as he stood up from his desk.

We reentered Bruce's exam room, and Dr. Brain sat on Bruce's level to deliver the news. "Bruce, I think I may know what is going on with you, and it's not good," he started. "Your symptoms and progression of your weakness and tremor lead me to a very bad diagnosis: ALS, or Lou Gehrig's disease. Have you heard of it?" he asked gently and sincerely.

"ALS?" Bruce's wife nearly shouted back at Dr. Brain as tears welled up in her eyes. "There's no way! No one in his family has this problem!"

Dr. Brain acknowledged her protest and returned his focus to the patient. "Bruce, we will need to do a variety of tests to confirm this diagnosis. It is rarely hereditary, and receiving this diagnosis is one that no one wants to hear. We caught it pretty early, so that is good news."

Bruce stared intently at Dr. Brain and looked like he had just seen a ghost. All color had drained from his face. "Tell me what I should expect from here," Bruce said in a quiet voice as his wife began to weep. The beautiful, polished middle-aged couple began to fall apart right in front of me. I felt uncomfortable and unnecessary at that moment.

"I wish I had better news to report. ALS is a progressive neurological disease that affects motor neurons - the nerves that allow your skeletal muscles to work. Your brain and spinal cord are essentially being attacked, causing your muscles to not work properly. The fact that your speech has been affected is also a worrisome sign, indicating the disease is progressing," Dr. Brain continued.

"How long do I have left to live?" Bruce asked point-blank while staring intently at Dr. Brain. Many physicians will avoid answering that question or beat around the proverbial bush, but Dr. Brain didn't mince words.

"After diagnosis, most people can live for years, but the average is around three years," he answered. "With the current advancements in medicine, you could live much longer. I will call the university hospital to see if they have any medication trials going on for ALS."

Bruce turned and looked at his wife and exclaimed, "What the fuck!"

I don't remember much else from the rest of Bruce's visit, as I was completely wrecked by his presumed diagnosis and their response. Dr. Brain concluded the interview by ordering bloodwork, an MRI, an electromyography (EMG), and nerve conduction studies. We finished up in the exam room and reconvened in Dr. Brain's office.

"Liz, this is my least favorite neurological diagnosis to deliver, but I try to always leave my patients with hope," he said. "This disease is more common in men, and hits them in the prime of their life. Medication can help a bit, but Bruce may be in a wheelchair in the not-too-distant future and may require a ventilator if he lives long enough. This diagnosis is always tragic, and usually happens to the nicest people, in my experience."

Dr. Brain's words left me feeling like I had been punched in the gut. I was overwhelmed at the thought of telling a once-healthy 55-year-old man that he couldn't expect a future with his family, and that the road ahead would be rocky. It was times like this that I seriously reconsidered medicine, not sure I could handle all of the devastating diagnoses. I realized that I needed to choose my future specialty carefully.

The rest of my rotation with Dr. Brain was filled with a more "garden variety" of neurological afflictions: strokes, multiple sclerosis, Parkinson's, and Alzheimer's disease. I learned a lot about this complex specialty and realized it was not for me; too many diseases with too little to offer afflicted patients.

I was grateful for my month of neurology training with such an incredible clinician, but thankful that I did not see any more patients with ALS in my rotation with Dr. Brain.

Chapter 8
Home Visit

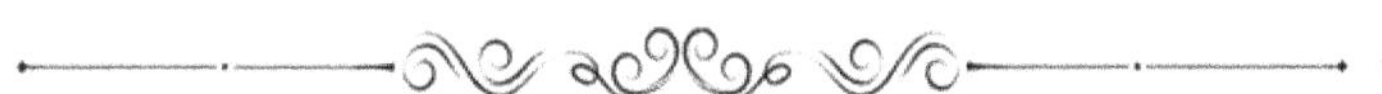

One of my rotations in medical school was outpatient pediatrics. As I already had one child and one on the way, I was excited to learn more about children and their afflictions. I was assigned to work with a well-known and well-loved pediatrician in a nice part of town. I was excited at the prospect of a civilized month of work in an outpatient pediatric setting.

On the first day of my rotation, I arrived at the office early and entered through the front entrance. Per usual, I was recognized by the staff as a medical student by my short, white coat.

"You must be Liz," a welcoming receptionist stated as I approached the desk. I noticed the bright colored animal murals on the walls, similar to those in the hospital. Approximately one-third of the waiting room was designated as a play area with copious toys scattered about. I wondered if they were remotely sanitary.

"Hi, yes. I'm Liz, here to work with Dr. Kid," I replied.

"Dr. Kid is in her office. You'll find her straight through this door at the end of the hall," she replied.

I entered the door labeled "private" and quickly found Dr. Kid, working at her desk. She was middle-aged and attractive, with a kind countenance.

"Hi, Dr. Kid, I'm Liz, your medical student for the month," I said as I entered her office and took a seat in a chair facing her.

"Hi, Liz. Rule #1 here: no white coat. We don't wear them as it can make children uncomfortable, so please hang your coat on the back of my door," she stated.

I listened to her unconventional introduction and obediently took off my coat. She wasn't rude, but she also wasn't necessarily nice. Initially, I wasn't sure what to expect from her, but what I quickly learned was that she was a woman of few words, and when she spoke, her words had meaning. Sometimes bluntness is just warranted, I surmised. But kindness did seem to be her general rule.

"We have a very full practice, Liz. Our days are exceptionally busy, and I also offer evening home visits to a few of my patients, when warranted," she said. "I know it's outside of traditional 'office hours,' but we may have a home visit while you are on your rotation this month. If we do, I would really like for you to join me if you can."

"I would be happy to join you at a patient's home," I replied without hesitation. As a medical student, you really aren't supposed to say no to your attending, regardless of what you are agreeing to.

"Great. Now let's go see our first patient," she said as she stood up from her desk and wrapped a stethoscope around her neck.

For the next two weeks, we worked together every day in her office, seeing innumerable patients with various diagnoses: colds and flu; well-child checks; vaccinations; ADHD; and more. Dr. Kid was an excellent teacher and mentor to me. When she learned of my child at home and child on the way, she spent extra time imparting her wisdom as we worked together. My time with her was a very civilized rotation, and I even considered pediatrics for myself.

Towards the end of my rotation with Dr. Kid, she let me know that she needed to see one of her patients at their home, and invited me to join her.

"Liz, we need to go see my patient, Mike, in his home. I've followed him for five years since his birth. His behavior has become so severe that his family would like me to see him in his home environment. We will leave as soon as we finish with our last patient today. We can drive together in my car," Dr. Kid finished.

"Sounds good," I replied. I borrowed Dr. Kid's landline and let my husband know I would not be home for dinner, or likely our child's bedtime.

After we had finished in the office for the day, Dr. Kid and I got into her Volvo and drove to meet Mike. He lived with his parents in the wealthiest suburb of our city. The drive into the family's neighborhood was inspiring and intimidating. Once we made it through the guarded gate, we weaved our way through the most opulent neighborhood I had ever seen in the city. Massive estates on manicured acres were the standard. Luxury vehicles and chauffeured limousines were the norm. I was impressed and wondered why Dr. Kid needed to do a home visit.

As we drove through the neighborhood, Dr. Kid said, "Liz, as you can tell, this family is *very* wealthy. The father, Mr. Smith, is a very successful businessman. He is married, with three children, all of whom see me as their pediatrician. Mike is their youngest, their only son, and the only child with a problem," she continued. "I'm not going to tell you what is wrong with Mike. You will soon see what this family is dealing with."

We pulled into the circular driveway of the Smiths' impressive estate and parked. Before we could ring the doorbell at the grand entrance, we were met at the front door by Mrs. Smith and her eight-year-old daughter.

"Hi, Dr. Kid, thank you so much for coming to our home," Mrs. Smith said as Dr. Kid and I entered the marble foyer. The house was so impressive that it took concentration not to stare at the opulence around me. From what I could see, the house looked like a museum.

"Hi, I'm Liz, a student doctor working with Dr. Kid," I offered as I held out my hand to Mrs. Smith. She shook my hand and gave me a warm, welcoming smile.

"Glad you could join us, Liz. My husband, Mike, and our younger daughter are in the basement. We would like to have the family meeting down there," she said as she turned around and started walking into the house. "Please follow me."

We all walked through the home to the entrance to the basement stairs near the kitchen. The home was incredible, with travel artifacts, original artwork, and expensive furniture everywhere you looked. The basement was somewhat of a misnomer, as the lower level was a continuation of the main floor grandeur. As we entered the beautiful subterranean area, we saw Mr. Smith and his daughter sitting on a gorgeous leather couch, reading a book together. I looked around the room and didn't see Mike.

Mr. Smith stood up and greeted us with a warm hello. "Thank you, Dr. Kid, for coming to our home. Things with Mike are not getting any better, and we really don't know what to do at this point," he offered.

"I understand. I'm glad we are here. Where is Mike?" Dr. Kid asked in reply.

"He's in the other room. He is on a time-out. I'll bring him in soon," Mr. Smith replied. "We can chat together until his time out is over."

At that very moment, a wiry, whirling dervish of a boy dressed only in his underwear flew into the main room where we were all sitting. Mike was holding an armful of stuffed animals and toys and proceeded to run around the room, throwing and scattering them everywhere. Mike's parents attempted to get him to calm down, but they couldn't.

It was at this point that I realized that Mike was completely non-verbal. Instead of speech, he offered grunts and shrieks to interact with his parents and Dr. Kid. He appeared to me to be completely out of control. In opposition to what his parents wanted him to do, Mike disappeared into the adjacent room and continued to shriek.

We took the opportunity to talk about Mike without further disruptions.

Dr. Kid and I sat with the parents as they discussed Mike and his ever-worsening behavior. He had been kicked out of both preschool and kindergarten for his behavioral issues, and this was now a significant problem for the family. Dr. Kid had diagnosed Mike with autism at age three, and his behavior had seemed to worsen every year since then. His parents were vocal and convinced that Mike's immunizations were to blame for his autism. Dr. Kid did not endorse that idea, but I listened to them without judgment. This was the first time I had heard of any link to autism from immunizations. It made me think of my own child and their shots.

As we continued to talk, Mike reappeared by running at full speed into the room, completely naked. He took his hands and began to smear a brown substance all over the walls of the room, which I assumed was finger paint. His parents continued our conversation and initially did not pay attention to Mike and his activities on the wall. Suddenly, and mid-conversation, Mike shrieked loudly and ran up to his mother and smacked his hands forcefully on both sides of her face. She recoiled from both the assault and from the substance he was smearing on her cheeks.

"Oh my God, Michael!" his mother shouted at him as she forcefully pulled his hands down from her face. Mike immediately grunted loudly and ran away to the adjacent room and hid. "He's smearing his shit everywhere! He's never done *this* before," Mrs. Smith finished as she got up to go attend to Mike and his mess.

Mr. Smith sat on the couch with his two daughters, and they all looked horrified and dejected. The girls started coughing from the smell of Mike's bowel movement. They got up and left to go upstairs, completely grossed out by their brother.

"Holy crap, Dr. Kid, pun intended. What are we supposed to do here?" Mr. Smith implored the professional sitting next to him on the sofa.

"Well, Mr. Smith, your son's behavior is certainly worsening, and what we witnessed tonight is a bad omen for future behavior," she replied honestly. "At this point, we need to involve a multidisciplinary team to help him. I will work on those arrangements when I get back to my office tomorrow," she finished.

At that point, Mrs. Smith reappeared with a bucket of sudsy water and a large sponge. She started to clean the poop off the walls. "I put Mike in the tub. I need to go get him cleaned up now. Thank you, Dr. Kid, for coming to our home," she finished. She looked completely disheartened.

Dr. Kid and I stood up and prepared to go upstairs to leave. I had a pit in my stomach, and I felt nauseated due to the circumstances and the odor. My heart was heavy at the thought of how this child's affliction was affecting his family. Gone were idyllic family vacations, sanguine family gatherings, and all hopes of a normal family life. No amount of money or success in the world could make up for what I had just witnessed in their mansion.

Back in the car, Dr. Kid started to impart her wisdom on autism. "It's a spectrum disease, Liz, and Mike is severely afflicted. As we saw tonight, even minor changes in his environment, like our arrival in his home, can cause extreme distress or meltdowns. I'd have to call the 'shit smearing' a meltdown," she said in a resigned tone. "He most likely has an IQ below 70 and has a dismal future ahead of him. He's going to need a lot of help, and his family is going to need respite care as well. He is a so-called 'lucky child' in that his parents have significant resources. The parents, not so lucky," she finished.

We drove in relative silence back to Dr. Kid's office so I could retrieve my car. I was heart-sick for what I had just witnessed in the Smiths' home. Seeing the pain and distress in their daughters' faces left a lasting impression on me. It was clear that the Smith family could no longer have a normal life with such an autistic child in the mix. I felt sadness and empathy for them.

My own child was asleep by the time I got home. My day's activities reminded me to hold my sleeping child in my arms until I fell asleep myself in the rocking chair. I didn't want to let go of my baby, and prayed that autism would stay far away from my own family.

Autism, or autism spectrum disorder (ASD), rates have continued to rise and now affect one in 30 children nationwide, and roughly one in 12 in California. Boys are diagnosed four times more often than girls. Approximately 27% of all autistic 8-year-olds are "profoundly" affected, meaning they are non-verbal, have severe behavioral issues, and poor outcomes. The research shows that environmental and genetic factors may contribute, but no definitive cause or treatment has been found. The vaccine theory continues to be debated.

Autism affects over 2% of our adult population, and roughly 20-30% of all autists are considered severe. Seventy-five percent of autists face under- or unemployment, putting strain on our entire system. Severe autism typically shows profound deficits in verbal and non-verbal communication; extreme sensitivity to sensory stimuli; repetitive behaviors; and limited ability to function independently. Most severely-afflicted autists require lifelong, intensive support and specialized care. As independent living is rarely feasible, many live in group home facilities or with family. Social isolation and caregiver burnout are significant issues.

Better awareness and early detection of autism, combined with early intervention and a multi-disciplinary approach, is now the standard of care.

Chapter 9
Binary Science

Most of us know that we live in a binary world: Hot/Cold. Up/Down. In/Out. Black/White. 0/1, etc.

But what about Boy/Girl? What about Man/Woman? What about XX/XY chromosomes?

Until very recently in our evolution as a species, we generally accepted that our genders were also binary. As a medical student in the early 1990s, I was taught that there are only two general, genetic genders, otherwise called your "genotype." But there are many ways to express that gender, known as your "phenotype."

The political debate regarding genders that is currently raging on seems to conflate these two scientific terms. Your genotype is assigned at conception when a sperm and egg combine to create a gender-defining set of chromosomes:

XX (female) or XY (male). While there are anomalous variances, most other combinations of chromosomes would not be compatible with life and usually result in a spontaneous abortion or stillbirth.

Once your genetic code is defined in the womb, there are an infinite number of ways that gender can be expressed - the phenotype. Even before our current societal fascination with gender came into full-blown existence, we can admit that not all men are the same, and not all women are the same. For starters, we all know men who are effeminate and masculine women. Your environment can also alter and influence the expression of your genetics, as it has for the gender-fluid or gender-dysphoric individual.

But, make no mistake. When a man decides to identify as a woman, or a woman as a man, this is a phenotypical change, not a genetic change of their chromosomes. While work is being done on changing one's genetic code, we are not presently altering the XX/XY birthright in any mainstream laboratory that I know of. We are, however, making significant, irreversible phenotypical changes in the operating room and pharmacy.

While in medical school, I was assigned again to the university's plastic surgery department for a month-long rotation. The chief of this particular rotation was a man with the nickname of "renegade" for his unorthodox approach to the specialty of gender-affirming care. Dr. Renegade was relatively new to our institution from the East Coast and brought with him a new, emerging surgical specialty: gender reassignment.

The goal for the rotation was to learn all I could about this novel approach to patient care. Due to the sensitive nature of these surgeries, time in the operating room with Dr. Renegade was really not an option for students. As such, most of my learning would be done in the library and on the wards with the patients pre- and post-transition. The patients undergoing gender reassignment were few and far between at that time, but their care was complex and required a lot of attention from the team pre- and post-surgery.

One morning, at our usual 7 a.m. meeting, Dr. Renegade addressed me specifically in the room full of students and residents. "Hey Liz, would you like to join me today in the operating room? We are surgically transitioning a man into a woman today."

I wasn't sure *why* I was being singled out, but I quickly said, "Absolutely."

"Perfect. Meet me in OR #9 in an hour," he finished as he left the room.

I looked around the cramped room of my colleagues and felt a bit sheepish. "Look who lucked out with facetime in the OR with Dr. Renegade," one of the other male students said in a sarcastic tone, to no one in particular. It was times like this that brought out the unnecessary competitiveness among the team. I decided against responding to my colleague and simply left the room myself.

I had no idea how long the surgery would be, so I took the opportunity to get some breakfast in the cafeteria and use the restroom. Then I put on OR scrubs and met Dr. Renegade at the scrub-in sink outside OR #9. "So, Liz, have you ever seen this type of operation?" he asked me as he moved the iodine sponge from his hands up his arms.

"No, sir," I replied. "I have heard of this surgery, have followed your patients post-op, but have never seen the surgery myself."

"Well, I invited you into my OR today because of the good work you have done with my patients on the wards. You will only be able to watch today. I may have you hold a retractor, *if* you're up for it," he shot back, sarcastically and with a smile.

Up for holding a retractor? Seriously? Of course, I can do that! I thought to myself as I remained quiet and continued scrubbing.

We entered the OR together and donned our sterile gowns, gloves, and hats with the help of a scrub nurse. The patient was already prepped and on the table. It looked as though he had been prepped for both "top" and "bottom" surgery. Dr. Renegade motioned for me to join him at the patient's groin.

"Liz, this is Mr. Miller, soon to be Ms. Miller," Dr. Renegade introduced me to the anesthetized patient as we gazed at his genitals peeking out from the sterile drapes. "He is 35 years old and has decided he is ready for the final stage of his transition. He has been on Lupron for years, and has been living as a woman for the past two years - a requirement of mine for this surgery," he replied. "In case you were wondering, I don't operate on anyone under the age of 25. Gotta have a fully formed cortex for my services."

Dr. Renegade continued, "Today, we are going to perform a procedure called 'penile inversion vaginoplasty.' Basically, I am going to create a vagina for *her* out of *his* penis and scrotum. When we are done 'downtown,' we will be giving her a beautiful set of boobs, 500cc of silicone per side. It's going to be a long procedure, so buckle up." My head was spinning at that point.

Dr. Renegade and I spent a total of eight hours together in the OR for the reassignment surgery. I watched with fascination - and a little horror - as he performed his work to turn male genitalia into something that really didn't approximate female genitalia at all. The most difficult part of the surgery seemed to revolve around creating a usable urethra, so she could pee.

Of secondary concern was a working vagina, which could also be addressed at a later surgery, if needed. Dr. Renegade said that Ms. Miller would need to use a "dilator" in her new vagina every single day of her life to avoid closure of the new vaginal tunnel. We finished our work "downtown," and changed out our gowns and gloves to move to the newly sterile and prepped "top surgery."

The breast augmentation surgery was the easiest procedure of all. Before we finished, Dr. Renegade admired his handiwork on Ms. Miller's breasts by sitting her up in the OR bed while still intubated and asleep.

"Looks good, huh, Liz?" he asked as he began to take off his gown and gloves, breaking the sterile field and indicating the surgery was over.

I wasn't really sure how to respond honestly. Yes, the large breast enhancement surgery was technically proficient, but seeing these huge silicone boobs on a 6'1" former man was a first for me. "I would say you did an excellent job, Dr. Renegade," I replied, knowing there really wasn't another answer to give.

"Liz, I'd like you to follow Ms. Miller while she is here in the hospital. Hopefully, she will be able to go home to her partner in about a week, if she doesn't need more surgery," he finished. I was glad that I would be able to follow her and agreed to the assignment.

I followed Ms. Miller for the three weeks she was hospitalized after her surgery. She had several post op complications, which can be expected with such an extensive surgery, but she was ultimately able to be discharged after she was able to pee without a catheter.

I met her partner, Johnathon, who seemed to be a loving and supportive person. Following the surgery, Ms. Miller's mood was what I would call "elated." This surgery was the final step in her decade-long goal of living openly as a woman. Her biggest hope was that she would no longer be misgendered as a man.

Before she left the hospital, Jonathon helped Ms. Miller fix her hair and put on makeup. He also brought her a beautiful, feminine pantsuit to wear at the time of discharge. I had to admit that she really was a beautiful woman. It was sad to see her go, and I acknowledged that it did seem to be the right procedure for her. It was satisfying to see her so happy. At that time, pronouns did not capture the public's fascination with gender-affirming care, and Ms. Miller was simply she/her.

Gender reassignment surgery benefits reportedly include reduced gender dysphoria, improved mental health, and increased self-esteem of the patient. Sexual function post-transition cannot be guaranteed, and many patients can no longer have an orgasm for the rest of their lives, post-transition. Unfortunately, these surgeries have a very high complication rate, and healing can take months. Sometimes, multiple surgeries are required, and expensive time away from work and family is required.

Of course, regret is the least desired outcome, and fortunately, it appeared at that time to be less common than satisfaction with the procedures. Costs for these surgeries are high and can range from $10,000-$50,000, depending on the procedures performed. In the 1990s, no insurance would cover this surgery, leaving the entire expense paid by the patient out of pocket.

At last check in 2025, there are now at least 78 gender-affirming pronouns that we are asked to embrace to describe two chromosomal genders. I think most of us can agree that this is an onerous number of pronouns to keep track of and to know intuitively who to address with each one.

Worse yet, there have been significant societal repercussions for using the incorrect pronoun, no matter if it is intentional or accidental; job losses, public ridicule, bullying, intimidation, etc. I am left to wonder *why* we have gotten to this point, not how.

Gender fluidity is common in childhood. I would submit that it is a normal rite of passage for most children. Most of us have witnessed little boys playing with dolls and little girls playing with trucks. Childhood is a time when children, without societal prejudice or pressure, can often act like the opposite sex or make comments about wanting to *be* the opposite sex. These comments and behaviors from children, in my humble opinion, should be met with indifference and a lack of judgment of that child. "Tincture of Time" is a fantastic treatment, and most children grow out of their gender-bending flights of fancy.

A more concerning aspect of this rampant gender dysphoria is why we are seeing so much of it. I believe it is the double-whammy of the pandemic of 2020 and social media. In the last several years, children have been distanced from societal norms and enveloped in a 24/7 web of undue influence by the corrupt social media companies, which promote gender confusion.

Recently, and within seconds of setting up a fake account for a 13-year-old girl on a popular social media platform, the account was flooded with porn, transgenderism, drug use, and violence. A child, no matter how sophisticated, cannot be expected to sift through this kind of material to know where their true compass reads.

So, children and adults, too, need to understand that chromosomal sex is scientifically binary. Expression of that gender is a phenotype - and includes medications, operations, makeup, and clothing.

Seventy-eight pronouns to describe these variations is simultaneously way too much and not enough.

Chapter 10

The VA

My next rotation was at the Veterans Administration (VA) medical center. To be honest, I had no idea what to expect. I had been told that doing internal medicine on a VA ward was one of the hardest rotations in all of medical school. The veteran patients can be so complex, with multiple medical problems and very often a challenging psychological overlay. The VA was a far cry from the other hospital wards and was intimidating to me, to say the least. The facility was huge and sterile, and the ancillary staff seemed to be chronically in short supply.

I arrived on my first day at 6:45 a.m. and took a seat in the tiny doctor's break room and waited for my colleagues. One by one, my fellow student doctor, intern, resident, and attending filed into the small room and took their seats. After brief introductions, our attending asked each of us to say a few words about ourselves.

Our attending started the introductions. He hailed from Boston and Harvard, and had an ego and arrogance to match his credentials. He made it clear that academic rigor was expected, and prolonged hours and no personal life were the standards of this month-long rotation. If he was trying to intimidate us, he accomplished his goal, and we all looked terrified to speak.

As we went around the room, giving our introductions, I listened as the group revealed their academic background, their hobbies, their favorite food, etc. When it was my turn, I gave similar information about myself, but added that I was a new mother and had recently returned from maternity leave. This information not only landed like a lead brick, but no one else in the room seemed to be able to relate to having children, including Dr. Harvard.

The only other medical student on this rotation was a young woman who had been in the class behind me before I took the extra year. She was younger than me, slender, beautiful, and dressed for work at the VA like she was going out on the town. Rather than be guided by Dr. Harvard to be more appropriate in her attire, the remaining of our colleagues - all men - chose to ogle at her 24/7, which she seemed to love. Every day, she sported a new sexy outfit and always styled her hair and put on makeup, in contrast to most other medical students in my school.

I, coming back from maternity leave, still had too many extra pounds on my body to dress like that (as if I even owned those clothes!) That first day, Jennifer's outfit with a plunging neckline and short skirt was in sharp contrast to my baggy, post-baby clothes. It didn't bother me that she looked fabulous all the time; it bothered me that the men on our service seemed to think that she was significantly more intelligent than I, as conferred by her appearance. Jennifer was given easier patient assignments and lavish praise by our attending for simply "doing her job."

Upon returning to medical school on this rotation at the VA, after having my child, I decided to continue to breastfeed my baby for a longer period than my six-week leave from medical school. I bought a breast pump, practiced with it, and brought it with me on my first day of work at the VA.

After our introductory morning meeting, the group broke up to go see our assigned patients. I approached Dr. Harvard with trepidation and asked him a verboten question.

"Excuse me, sir, I need to pump breast milk while I am on this rotation. Can you direct me to where I can do that?" I asked.

Dr. Harvard looked at me in horror, as if I had asked him to give up his prestigious position and credentials.

"Excuse me? Breastfeed?" he asked in disbelief and with a disgusted look on his face.

"Yes, I will need to take 10 minutes twice a day. Is there a place I can go to do that?" I asked again.

"Liz, we don't have time for extracurricular activities like that on this service. You will have to find another option," he replied.

Another option? What the hell does that mean? Stop breastfeeding my child at six weeks? I wondered. I couldn't believe what I was hearing, but I wasn't surprised. Dr. Harvard had a reputation that preceded him, that of a hardass and an asshole. He certainly was living up to that reputation with this interaction with him.

"I see," I responded, while keeping my composure, when all I really wanted to do was scream something very unkind at him.

Dr. Harvard had clearly decided our conversation about breastfeeding was done and quickly left the room, as if he was fleeing a contagious disease. It was apparent that I had made him *very* uncomfortable by discussing breastfeeding. I decided it was none of his business what I did with my two 10-minute breaks in a 24-hour period of work, and I was sorry that I had asked him to begin with.

True to his answer, there really wasn't anywhere at the VA to respectfully and privately pump breast milk, so I cowered in a dirty bathroom stall and pumped to keep up my milk supply. Unfortunately, I had to dump it out each time because the VA wouldn't allow me to store it anywhere in refrigeration. It felt like a hostile work environment.

After my initial unpleasant conversation with Dr. Harvard, I did not discuss my private life with him again, and I'm sure he thought he had talked me out of continuing to breastfeed my newborn child. I had learned on day one of working with him to keep my mouth shut.

My weeks at the VA were agonizing and difficult. The patients were indeed very complex, but they were also the best adult patients I have ever worked with. The men and the women - mostly men at the VA at that time - were incredible people who often were suffering injuries and illnesses caused by their service to our country's freedom. It was humbling, shocking, and terrifying to learn of their tours and their lives once home. Truly a life-changing experience for me. So rewarding when you can offer help to them; devastating when they succumb to their illnesses.

One day, I had a little extra time on my hands, and I decided to join one of my patients for a colonoscopy that I had ordered, suspecting colon cancer. As was required at the time, the physician performs a digital rectal exam (DRE) before inserting the scope. This attending, whom I had never met before, thought it would be "fun" for *me* to do the DRE on our patient, the first of my life.

The GI attending physician instructed the patient to bend over the stretcher and present his bare ass to me. He did so, but when he realized that I would be performing the rectal exam, not the male attending, he flipped out. He stood up straight, turned around, and faced me directly and said, "Lady, when I bend over and see shoes, they better be only 'wing-tips!'" This meant he would only accept a prostate exam from someone of his gender, with the appropriate shoes.

I totally understood where he was coming from, and didn't mind the idea that he didn't want me to perform the DRE exam anyway. I did, however, purchase a pair of Doc Martens wing-tip shoes the next day, and wore them for the remainder of my time at the VA.

My rotation at the VA finally came to an end, and I was glad to give up the 100-hour work weeks with Dr. Harvard. He continued to shower Jennifer with attention, extra teaching, and praise, while I remained relatively ignored. I didn't think much of it until I received my grade for the rotation: a "D". I was in shock.

One-hundred-hour work weeks and sleeping at the hospital 3-4 nights a week away from my family; completion of every requirement; and excellent work with my patients, had come to this: overt sexual discrimination. I was stunned as this was the most blatant discrimination I had experienced up to that point in medicine.

The first thing I did after receiving my grade was to call Jennifer to ask her what her grade was: an "A"; shocker there. Second, I made an appointment with the dean's office (a different one from Dean Rude). I explained what had happened at the VA about my grade and the discrimination I had faced. I had to file a formal complaint and go through an investigation, but in the end, the grade was changed to accurately reflect the exceptional work that I had done.

Not too long afterwards, Dr. Harvard was sent back to the East Coast.

Chapter 11
Kai

My first day back in medical school after my second maternity leave did not go well. The school had apparently emailed me to tell me where to go and when to arrive for my community hospital rotation. But they sent it to the wrong student, so I never got the email.

When I arrived at the hospital on the second day of the rotation, alliances and favoritism were already determined, and I was clearly considered the outcast on the service. My rotation was inpatient pediatric gastroenterology, which I thought sounded cool, as I was a new mother. Little did I know that it would be one of the hardest rotations of my life.

A day in the life at the hospital - whether you are a student or an attending - starts at 7 a.m. sharp, sometimes earlier depending on the specialty. On my first day of the rotation, I grabbed a cup of crappy coffee from the nurse's station and took a seat in the tiny work room at 6:59 a.m., where "pre-rounds" occur. Meaning, the team of attending physicians, doctors in residency, and student doctors meet to discuss the patients on the census and make a plan for the day.

Many people think that the life of a doctor is somehow glamorous, but most of the time, it is just a ton of sometimes-rewarding work. Grunt work. Scut work. Call it whatever you want, it's *hard* work. And, "hard" can mean a lot of different things. Way more than simply the exhaustion that comes from working 80-100 hours a week. Hard includes losing patients to the grips of death, harassment, hazing, and "shit-rolls-downhill" attitudes. As you train and move up the medical ladder, you also hear a lot of "I had to suffer, so you have to suffer" type philosophy from your higher-ups.

Learning to be a good doctor is brutal. Interestingly, doctors-in-residency and student doctors are now limited to only 80 hours of work per week, but that limitation didn't exist when I was going through training. I realize saying "only 80 hours" could sound condescending, but those kinds of hours are expected in medicine.

Our team on the specialty pediatrics rotation was small, which meant "more learning" for those of us who were there. More learning also meant more work, but I was undeterred. I felt rested, invigorated, and ready to conquer my first rotation back after maternity leave. The attending physician, a most unpleasant, gruff, and condescending man, entered the room at 7:00 a.m. sharp and quickly addressed me.

"Liz, where were you yesterday?" the attending asked in front of the others in an accusatory tone.

I glanced around the room and apologized to everyone that I had missed the first day, a major no-no in medicine, with *very* few acceptable excuses. I started to explain my absence due to the administrative error, but our boss cut me off mid-sentence.

"Hopefully you've figured out your schedule and will improve from here," he shot back, clearly attempting to intimidate me. *Welcome to the first day of a new rotation in medical school,* I thought to myself.

I sat quietly as our attending, Dr. Rude, took his seat across from me and began to read the census. Most of the pediatric patients were a "garden variety" of pediatric gastroenterology hospital admissions: dehydration, inflammatory bowel disease, abdominal pain, etc. He then came to a new patient on the list.

"Let's see here," he said as he lifted his gaze from the census list and stared directly at me. "Liz, I want you to take this new admission and come see me after you've completed your history and exam," he said. "Let's see how good you are. This kid is a true medical mystery."

Dr. Rude continued, "This kid's parents are pot-smoking hippies from a rural area and are neglecting their child. He is six years old, and his primary care physician diagnosed him with failure to thrive (FTT). Let's see if you can figure this out. I've got him scheduled already for an upper endoscopy and a colonoscopy as soon as he arrives at the hospital and you are finished with his intake and admission note."

As Dr. Rude gave me the assignment, I froze in my seat and wondered if I was being punished for missing the prior day of work. I truly had no idea how to go about what I was being asked to do, and did not feel comfortable clarifying anything with him, especially in front of the group. It was my first clinical rotation in a pediatric hospital and my first experience as a "baby-doc" - pun intended - in pediatric gastroenterology.

I decided the best thing to do would be to simply spend time with the child and his family, take a really good history, and perform a thorough physical exam. I figured the rest would take care of itself in due time. I was grateful that Dr. Rude had given me the tip about the workup he had planned for this patient, as it gave me a starting place for his admission note and orders that I would ultimately write for him.

The little boy had been admitted to the GI service and was scheduled upon admission (before anyone had even laid eyes on him) for the upper and lower GI scope - two very invasive procedures requiring general anesthesia. My attending physician had let me know that my role was to basically confirm the working diagnosis and workup that he had already determined and planned, before ever seeing the patient.

I grabbed my requisite clipboard, stack of blank paper, and beeper. I wrapped my stethoscope around the neck of my short, white student coat and began to look for the patient's room. I only had two hours before the team would reconvene and perform "proper rounds" on all of the patients on our service.

"Rounding" means that the entire team - doctors, nurses, physical therapists, occupational therapists, and social workers - meet in a circle in the hallway outside the door of the patient to be discussed. The attending physician usually runs the rounds and calls on the students to do most of the talking, or hazing, as the case may be. This would mean that I had to not only examine my patient, but I had to come up with a care plan to present at rounds.

I approached my patient's hospital door and knocked gently as I peered in through the window and slowly opened it. I saw a young couple sitting on the bed with the mother holding their child in her arms. I approached the family and introduced myself, and instantly felt fear and horror, for unknown reasons.

"Hi, I'm Liz, a medical student here. I have been asked to speak with you and examine your son," I said with as much of a compassionate smile and false confidence as I could muster. The child curled up in front of me in his mother's arms was tiny, appearing to be only three or four years old, certainly meeting the criteria for FTT. He was emaciated and very pale. I reached out to touch his blonde hair and asked him in a soft voice, "Hi sweetie, what is your name?"

The little boy didn't answer me, but lifted his head off his mother's chest, with effort, and gave me a half smile before he flopped his head back down. His mother looked at me directly and said, "His name is Kai. We named him after the ocean in Hawaii, where we love to surf. It's also where Kai was conceived."

"That is a beautiful name," I replied, with tears welling up as I noticed Kai's resemblance to my own child. "Please tell me everything you can about your son and when things changed for him," I said as I pulled up a chair and sat on the parents' level.

My attending physician had reported to me that the family was poor and had not been feeding their son. He was very derogatory when describing the home environment, as conveyed to him by Kai's remote pediatrician. Even though he had not seen the home himself, he repeatedly said that the parents were "hippies" and were neglecting their parental responsibilities. Basically, he implied that Kai's parents were starving him to death.

The parents sitting before me on the bed really didn't seem to fit the typical description of deadbeat parents. Both of them were dressed well in expensive-looking clothes, shoes, and watches. They were well-groomed and seemed very attentive to their son. I did a little social sleuthing and learned that his parents were both engineers with master's degrees who worked in agriculture and farming in their rural town. At that point, I was even more determined to solve the mystery of Kai's illness, as the picture painted by Dr. Rude really didn't seem to be adding up.

Another indication that all was not as it appeared to be, as reported by the rural pediatrician, was the fact that the parents were excellent historians. Most often, if a child is being abused or neglected, the story relayed is never clear or without inconsistencies. Kai's story, as told by his parents, was precise, understandable, and shocking. They remembered dates with accuracy and put together an invaluable timeline of events for me in Kai's young life.

Kai's mother had a normal, uncomplicated pregnancy, and he was born at full term and without problems. For the first few years of his life, Kai had had a normal childhood, meeting all of his milestones. He was an only child and the light of his parents' lives. The more I learned from Kai's parents about his little life, the more concerned and alarmed I became.

Kai's story was tragic. Approximately two years earlier, at age four, Kai had started to eat less, becoming more of a picky eater by the day. He lost weight and began to lose interest in everyday activities suitable for a child his age. Eventually, he had lost so much weight that he had stopped most physical activities and had to drop out of Kindergarten due to his lack of energy. He had also lost the ability to focus and stay on task for even the most menial of activities in the classroom.

Kai's parents had taken him to a pediatrician in the rural area where they lived. He had seen Kai over the years and had come to develop his opinion of Kai's family. He believed that they were causing this harm to their son by their lifestyle (people who loved to surf and, admittedly, occasionally smoked pot). He had finally sent Kai to us in the "big city" in a fit of desperation. He did this to please the parents he had contempt for, having given up on Kai himself.

Basically, in a display of frustration, Kai's pediatrician had "dumped" him on our pediatric gastroenterology service, and it was now *my* job to think about what to do next. I tried to forget Dr. Rude's presumed diagnosis and pre-planned invasive workup. I approached Kai and his parents with neutrality, to avoid bias in my *own* assessment and proposed workup of Kai.

All I knew at that point was that these parents were incredibly distressed about the condition of their child and how they had been treated by the medical establishment thus far. I couldn't imagine what it would be like to have an ailing child and be so judged and dismissed by the medical system. I was shocked at what I was being told by Kai's parents, and I was determined to be a better provider of care to this beautiful child in front of me.

After taking a thorough history from his parents with an accurate timeline of Kai's illness, it was now time to turn my attention to Kai's physical exam. I performed everything I could while Kai rested in his mother's arms. Everything seemed to be fine: heart, lungs, abdomen, etc.

I then asked Kai's mom if I could see him walk. In response, she looked terrified. She let me know that Kai had lost the ability to walk over the past few months. I couldn't believe what I was hearing. *LOST his ability to walk at age six months ago - and we are now just seeing this child in referral?* I nearly said out loud.

My heart sank and began to beat very fast as I knew I had to see Kai walk or at least attempt to. Kai's mom did her best to try to dissuade me from making her son ambulate, knowing it might upset him. But I knew I had to make him at least try. I knew that I would glean *a lot* of information by seeing Kai move by himself.

At this point, I was thinking of many other diagnoses than Kai's gastrointestinal tract. His symptoms and progression of his illness, as reported by his parents, caused me to turn my attention to his neurological status. Watching Kai walk could elucidate a trove of information for me to ponder.

I reached out my hands and gently lifted Kai, who only weighed 35 pounds at that point, into my arms. I held him gently before slowly lowering his feet to the floor. When his bare feet touched the floor, Kai's legs started to shake vigorously as he attempted to steady himself. He grabbed onto me for dear life. After a minute or so, Kai was steady enough to stand in front of me unassisted.

"I can't believe he is standing by himself!" Kai's mom exclaimed excitedly. "He hasn't done that for months!"

"He's probably just showing off for me, Mom," I replied and smiled at her, trying to hide my alarm and dismay. Something really bad was going on with this child, and it was my job to try and figure out what was going on as soon as possible.

I stepped back about two feet from Kai while holding his outstretched arms and asked him to walk toward me. Before he moved, he gave me a huge, crooked smile and tilted his head all the way down to his right shoulder. He walked slowly and awkwardly toward me, only able to take a couple of very unsteady steps. He walked with an unbalanced gait, and as he did so, his eyes rolled up into his head.

"Mom and Dad, when did Kai start walking like this, with his head cocked to the side?" I asked as I tried to contain my outrage.

"About a year ago," his mom replied. "When we told his pediatrician that he couldn't walk without tilting his head, he said that Kai was doing it on purpose, to get attention. He said Kai probably saw someone walking this way on TV, and is trying to imitate him," she said.

"Has he seen anyone else besides your pediatrician?" I asked, hoping he had referred Kai to an outpatient specialist before this admission.

"No, he said he wasn't concerned. He said Kai would grow out of it," she finished.

I carefully picked Kai up and placed him gently back in his mother's arms. "Thank you so much for spending your time with me and telling me everything you did about Kai. You have been incredibly helpful. I will be back after I meet with my team," I said before leaving the room.

I shut the door behind me, took a deep breath, and wiped the tears from my eyes. I was shaking and had a pit in my stomach as I began to look for my attending. I found him playing a video game in the same office where we had met earlier. "Sir, I'd like to speak with you before we round," I said to Dr. Rude.

"What is it, Liz?" he asked in an irritated tone and with a sigh. "Do you have your admission note written for me yet?"

"Sir, I don't believe that my patient needs a GI workup. I believe he has a brain tumor," I blurted out.

At that point, Dr. Rude stopped playing his game and turned to look at me directly. "How about this: you stick to being a medical student, and I'll stick to being an attending physician. I have no use for your ridiculous diagnoses, I told you he is here for a GI workup!" he snapped at me.

Summoning up all the courage I could, I said, "Sir, I really don't think he needs a GI workup, but I think he really does need an MRI of his brain," I continued.

I realized that my recommendation to change course would be taking a significant amount of money out of his personal pocket if we swapped the GI workup for the brain MRI. I decided to change my tactic. "Perhaps we could order an MRI of his brain *in addition* to your planned workup?" I asked, hoping he would agree to the compromise.

"You can keep your erroneous opinions to yourself. I already told you why he is here and what I have scheduled for him," Dr. Rude finished and turned back to his computer game, indicating the conversation was over.

I felt a flood of emotions coursing through my body, and my face flushed red as I turned around and left the room. I hadn't written my admission note yet, and now I wasn't sure if I should stick to my story and put it in writing in the medical chart. Such a dilemma: stay true to my observations and probable clinical acumen, even as a medical student, or protect the attending physician and simply write a confirmatory GI admission note for him.

It is times like these that medical training can be dicey. As the lowest person on the doctor totem pole, I risked ridicule or even worse, a reprimand, if I deviated from my attending's plan for Kai. I decided that I would stick to my guns and write what I thought the diagnosis most likely was, Dr. Rude be damned. If I was wrong, no harm, no foul. They could blame me for a stupid note, written by a misguided and overzealous medical student. If I were right, I just might be able to help this beautiful child.

During rounds, I presented Kai's case to the group and gave my opinion of the workup I believed was needed. Dr.

Rude glared at me during the entirety of the meeting, but did not humiliate me further, and in public at that moment. Dr. Rude finished my case presentation of Kai by saying to the group, "Thank you, medical student number two. I will be scoping this patient later today. He is getting a full GI workup and won't leave this hospital until we have done every test possible for his gut issues that are causing his failure to thrive." I kept quiet about the fact that I had not found a single reason to work Kai up for gastrointestinal issues.

Because Kai was now "my patient" for the duration of his stay, or the end of my rotation, whichever came first, I followed him for the next couple of weeks. The planned GI workup - of course - was negative. As was a plethora of blood tests, ultrasounds of his abdomen, X-rays, CT scan of his abdomen, swallowing study, and more. He had an NG tube placed and had been receiving artificial nutrition and hydration.

Finally, after two weeks of hospitalization without any GI findings, a new attending physician rotated onto our service, replacing Dr. Rude. "Liz, what's going on with the kid in room #505?" he asked me one day before rounds.

"His name is Kai, and he's here for failure to thrive. He's had every test imaginable for that, but what he really needs is an MRI of his brain," I said confidently, ever more convinced that I was right. "I believe he has a brain tumor, sir," I finished.

"Yes, I read your excellent admission note. Please order an MRI with contrast of his brain," he finished. "It's time to get to the bottom of what is going on. This family deserves answers."

Kai's MRI came back with tragic findings. He had a tumor - later found to be a Glioblastoma Multiforme (GBM) - the size of a lemon at the base of his skull. Surgery was not an option due to the tumor's size and location. GBM is the deadliest form of brain cancer and confers a terrible prognosis. Kai was no exception, and he never left the hospital.

I was able to stay with Kai, rounding every day on him, and was even able to sit by his side with his family as he transitioned to the afterlife. Kai's parents and I had become quite close over the weeks, and they saw me as their only lifeline in a hostile medical establishment.

Kai's parents asked me to speak at his funeral, but I declined. I was so traumatized by the loss of Kai - juxtaposed with going home to my own beautiful tow head every evening that I didn't have to sleep at the hospital. I just knew I wouldn't make it through a single sentence without bawling.

I did go to Kai's funeral - an activity that is rarely done by a medical provider for their patient. Kai was different. This was personal. All I could think of that day - as I sat in the back row of the church and sobbed - was how Kai's early death may not have had to happen. If the medical establishment had replaced its judgment and discrimination with compassion and intellectual acumen, Kai could have been with us longer. This six-year-old soul should not have died that young.

Tragically, physicians and the medical system can be so biased and off-base at times.

Chapter 12
A Bad Birth

In my fourth year of medical school, and after I had given birth to my second child, I was assigned to the OBGYN service at the university hospital. Given that my rotation was only one month long, I knew I wouldn't be able to follow any patient for their whole pregnancy. Rather, I would be seeing a mix of patients at various stages of pregnancy, combined with live births, C-sections, and gynecologic issues. My time would be spent in the clinic, the operating room, and the hospital.

My first day on the service gave me a good insight into the month ahead that awaited me. I arrived on time at the clinic and walked into a full waiting room. Women, in various stages of pregnancy, filled every available chair. Some with partners, some alone. The receptionist noticed my short white coat and greeted me. "Hi, you must be our new student doctor," she said in a welcoming tone.

"Hi, yes, I'm Liz, your student for the month," I replied. "I'm here to work with Dr. Baby."

"Dr. Baby is at the hospital right now performing an emergency C-section. She will be back soon," the receptionist stated. "Her office is at the end of the hall. Please go there to wait for her."

I entered through the door labeled "private" and found Dr. Baby's office. The walls were covered with diplomas and awards, signifying her credentials and proficiency as a physician. The walls were intended to impress, and they did. I also noticed that her entire office was devoid of any family photos or personal mementos, unusual for a physician. I wondered if she ever had a reason to go home.

In preparation for this rotation, I had spoken with several student colleagues who had rotated on this service before me. I was told that the month would be a chaotic mix of scheduled office patients, GYN procedures, planned hospital births, C-sections, and emergency births. Babies rarely stick to planned timelines and have a nasty habit of being born at many inopportune moments: the middle of the night, weekends, and holidays. Due to this, the life of an OBGYN physician at that time was rarely smooth and predictable.

At that time, the specialty attracted a difficult personality type that could thrive in the professional chaos.

I was warned that I should mirror the attending physician's schedule as much as possible, without complaint or request for any special accommodation. I realized that I would see very little of my own family over the next 30 days and braced myself for a long, arduous month.

One of the most often discussed topics regarding physicians revolves around the concept of "bedside manner," a doctor's attitude or approach to a patient. In my tenure as a medical student, I had witnessed many different bedside manners from my teachers.

Generally, and in my personal experience by then, women and primary care physicians seemed to have the best bedside manners. But they would often avoid telling their patients the brutal truth about their diagnosis, instead preferring to leave their patients with hope. Surgeons generally, and some men specifically, had the worst bedside manner and didn't seem to care how the message they delivered was received by the patient.

I assumed that a female OBGYN physician, giving care to pregnant women giving birth to their baby, would be a shining example of a physician with great bedside skills. Boy, was I ever wrong.

My primary boss for the OBGYN rotation was an anorexically thin, six-foot-tall woman named Dr. Baby. She was middle-aged, single, and ironically, she didn't have any children of her own. She had the reputation of being very difficult to work with, requiring long hours with little feedback. My colleagues who had previously worked with her had warned me of the rigorous schedule and the generally unacknowledged work of underlings such as me. I wondered what awaited me, but didn't have to wait for long.

About an hour later, Dr. Baby flew into her office, briefly said hello to me, then instructed me to follow her into one of the overflowing exam rooms. We raced down the hall and checked the next patient's chart as we stood outside exam room #5. "Liz, this is a prenatal visit for this patient. She reports that she is around 16 weeks pregnant. She usually sees my partner for GYN issues, so this is her first prenatal visit, and this is the first time I am meeting her today."

Dr. Baby loudly knocked on the exam room door, and we entered the room together. "Hi Carrie, I'm Dr. Baby, and this is Liz, a medical student working with me." The patient was sitting on the exam table, and Dr. Baby and I took our seats in the room.

Dr. Baby flipped through Carrie's paper chart and confirmed the 16-week pregnancy. "Carrie, we need to talk. Your weight puts you in danger of a difficult pregnancy. I only want you to gain 10 pounds for the rest of your pregnancy. You can consider your pregnancy as a 'weight loss program,'" she stated directly and firmly. Her words sounded like a command to me.

I was shocked at what I was hearing, especially having had two pregnancies of my own. Carrie appeared to me to be of normal body weight, a fact I confirmed later in her chart. Carrie herself looked surprised and disheartened at the blunt and unusual dictate. "But, I thought I was *allowed* to gain weight if I'm pregnant," she protested.

Dr. Baby replied by simply stating, "Carrie, you're fat." The comment, said by someone of authority that you could call anorexic, left a sting in the air. I felt very uncomfortable in that moment and felt empathy for Carrie. You could feel Carrie's disappointment and discomfort. *What a buzz kill! Way to take the joy out of pregnancy,* I thought.

At this point, I had a pretty good idea of what Dr. Baby's bedside manner would be like. I was horrified at what she told Carrie, and couldn't imagine what I would have said and thought if my own OBGYN had told me the same thing during my pregnancies.

Additionally, I later did my own research in the library and could not find any medical recommendations for dieting during pregnancy. In fact, weight loss during pregnancy is rarely recommended, especially in a normal-weight person. Most pregnant women are advised to gain weight to support the baby's growth. Typically, 25-35 pounds over nine months if the mother has a normal BMI, like Carrie.

In fact, not gaining enough weight during pregnancy can increase risks of low birth weight, preterm delivery, or nutrient deficiencies for both the mother and baby. Of course, Dr. Baby and I did not ever discuss this issue, and she did not ever explain her reasoning to me for lecturing Carrie about her weight.

The rest of my first day with Dr. Baby flew by. We saw a punishing schedule of patients in the clinic, skipped lunch to fit in a few more patients, and ended our day by rounding on her hospitalized patients. Twelve hours of following her around like a puppy as she raced through her day; no food or breaks, and little teaching. I arrived home at nearly 9 p.m., exhausted with my head spinning. I held and kissed my sleeping children briefly before falling into bed myself.

The remainder of my month pretty much mirrored my first day. I found the chaotic OBGYN specialty to be antithetical to the type of practice I wanted for myself. One day, toward the end of my rotation with Dr. Baby, she sat me down in her office to discuss a difficult case before we left for the hospital.

"Liz, I've got a patient in active labor at the hospital. She seems to be okay, but her child is in distress and is being closely monitored. I may need to do an emergency C-section. Change into scrubs and meet me in the maternity ward as soon as possible," Dr. Baby barked as she stood up from her desk and headed for the door.

The hospital wasn't within walking distance, so I drove myself there and changed into hospital scrubs. I walked to the maternity ward and asked for Dr. Baby's whereabouts. "Excuse me, can you tell me where Dr. Baby is?" I asked the receptionist at the nurse's station.

"Dr. Baby is attending to the patient in room #909. There's pretty high drama in there right now. You might want to wait a bit," the lady offered, perhaps trying to protect me from the goings-on in the patient's room. I knew that I was more likely to get in trouble if I *didn't* go into the room, so I thanked the receptionist for her information and entered the room quietly.

Dr. Baby was standing over the bed, watching the baby's "decels" on a monitor next to the bed. Decels are a worrisome slowing of the baby's heart rate, indicating the baby is in distress. The mother, lying in bed, appeared terrified. Flashes of my own pregnancies and deliveries raced through my mind as I oriented myself to what was going on. I stood at the foot of the bed and waited to be introduced.

"Liz, this is Stephanie. She is 36 weeks pregnant and has had a normal pregnancy until about a month ago, when her baby stopped gaining weight. Her baby is not happy at the moment. His heart rate decreases significantly with each one of her pre-term contractions. If this continues, she is buying herself an emergency C-section," she divulged in front of Stephanie. "We will know more in the next hour." Stephanie started to cry, and Dr. Baby did nothing to console her.

I wasn't sure what to do at that point, so I decided to stay with Stephanie as we waited for Dr. Baby's decision. Over the next hour, and after a few more dramatic decelerations of the baby's heart rate, Dr. Baby decided to liberate him from his hostile environment.

Once the emergency C-section was authorized, the mayhem really began. The patient and bed were rushed by the nurses to the nearby operating room located within the maternity ward. The team surrounding the bed listened to the orders shouted out to them by Dr. Baby, as they moved the bed down the hall as fast as they could. When we reached the OR, the ballet began at warp speed. Sterile drapes, anesthesia, a baby monitor, and more were put into place at a rapid pace. Per custom at the time, the pregnant patient herself was not allowed to see her baby being born by C-section, as the sterile drapes blocked the view.

I scrubbed into the sterile OR and joined Dr. Baby at Stephanie's abdomen. She didn't acknowledge me or hand me a retractor, so I just stood there and watched. I could tell that she was stressed out and understood that I had little to offer her at that point. Rapidly, she skillfully exposed the distressed baby and brought his blue body out of Stephanie's womb. "Liz, we've got a big problem here, the umbilical cord is wrapped around his neck," Dr. Baby reported. I wasn't sure what she was implying, so I summoned up the courage to ask.

"Can you fill me in, Dr. Baby?" I asked genuinely, not sure if the baby was alive or not, as I viewed his lifeless body.

"I don't have time for your ignorance; this baby is in trouble!" she shot back in front of the whole team in the OR.

Yikes! Note to self: Stay quiet, no matter what! I thought to myself as I watched Dr. Baby pull out the cyanotic newborn from Stephanie's womb.

"Shit! Call the neonatologist on call! We need help here," Dr. Baby shouted to the charge nurse. At that point, I backed away from the operating table to give the team more room to work. It became clear that Stephanie's baby was indeed in great distress, if he was alive, and my presence there was not needed or welcomed.

The baby was taken to a nearby table where the team worked to get him to breathe. Stephanie, hidden behind the sterile drape, was awake and crying to see her newborn. The tension in the air in that OR could have been cut with a knife. I watched as Dr. Baby and her team attempted to revive the baby. It did not look like it was going well. Dr. Baby shouted at a weeping Stephanie, "Stephanie, stop wailing! We are trying to save your son!" With that comment, I began to feel ill.

A neonatologist quickly appeared in the OR and joined in the resuscitation effort. In the end, the attempts to save the baby were not successful. Once the decision was made to stop the resuscitation protocol, the deceased baby was quickly placed on Stephanie's chest.

I watched in horror as she loudly wept, and the team began to clean up the OR around her. They performed their tasks quickly and quietly while ignoring Stephanie and the dead infant in her arms. It felt surreal. I walked to the head of the bed and addressed Stephanie myself. "I know I can't do anything but say I'm so sorry," I said as tears flowed down her face.

"Liz! Time to go!" Dr. Baby barked at me. She hadn't even spoken a kind word to Stephanie when I followed her out of the OR.

"How often does this happen, Dr. Baby?" I asked her as we raced down the hospital corridor, heading back to her office to see more patients.

"It happens. That's life. She can get pregnant again," she replied callously.

I was shocked at her response and felt like I needed to throw up. I couldn't wait to rotate off of Dr. Baby's service. Fortunately, this episode occurred late in my month-long rotation with her, and I didn't witness any more neonatal deaths.

Chapter 13
Seizure Boy

In my fifth year of medical school, I was assigned to an inner city hospital on the pediatric neurology service. As I had two children of my own by then, I was excited to learn about what kinds of neurological problems I would find in children. Because I was the only medical student on the service, I would have lots of "facetime" with my attending physician, Dr. Maverick. It also meant that there would be lots of work for me to do, and I consoled myself with the fact that I would also learn a lot.

After my experience with Kai, I had somewhat of a perverse interest in this subject that could affect my own two children. A pursuit of knowledge "by proxy."

I arrived extra early for my first day. I weaved my way through the hospital to the pediatric wing, always bright and sunny with colorful murals on the hall walls. I wondered if the attempt to bring cheer actually provided any value, or if these murals were the result of ideas conceived in boardroom meetings. *Do the ill children even notice the walls? Do they make any difference?* I wondered.

Regardless, the entrance to the ward was decidedly cheerful. I walked towards the nearest nurses' station and asked for the whereabouts of Dr. Maverick. "Hello, I'm a new medical student working on the pediatric neurology service. Do you know where I am supposed to meet the team?" I asked.

"Dr. Maverick has an office just down this hallway on the left," a nice nurse responded. "He is waiting for you there."

I quickly found the office and introduced myself to my new boss for the next month. "Hello, my name is Liz, I'm your medical student on this rotation." He held out his hand, and I shook it before sitting down in the tiny room that looked like a closet, except for the two computers.

Dr. Maverick was not young, but he also wasn't old. He had hair like Einstein, and his clothes were disheveled under his wrinkled and stained white lab coat. He had a kind face and a pleasant countenance. He was highly regarded nationally in his specialty, but was known as somewhat of an oddball non-conformist in his approach to certain pediatric diseases. I was excited to learn from him.

"Tell me about yourself, Liz," Dr. Maverick stated as I sat down.

"Well, I'm in my last year of medical school, I'm married, and I've had two children over the past couple of years," I replied. "I'm looking forward to being on this service."

"Well, you may not be excited for long," he replied. "We see lots of very sick children on this service. What we will see is not common, so don't worry about your own children. We only see the worst of the worst in this hospital." I wasn't sure if I should be comforted or terrified.

As we finished our conversation, two residents entered and sat on the two remaining chairs in the tiny room. We introduced ourselves to each other and waited for instructions from Dr. Maverick.

"Well, team, we have a new medical student, as you can see, and I am going to give her only the toughest patients," Dr. Maverick said as he looked at me with a mischievous grin. This kind of comment from the attending was expected as a student and part of the usual hazing that occurs in medicine. But when Dr. Maverick said it, it seemed a bit more benign than the previous attendings. I wasn't sure what he meant by the "toughest patients" but I knew enough to simply smile in return, giving my tacit approval for the upcoming assignments.

"Liz, we have a new patient coming in this morning, and I'd like you to be his primary provider, reporting directly to me," Dr. Maverick offered. "He is coming from far away in the state and should be here in a couple of hours. He is four years old with intractable seizures. Why don't you spend the morning researching pediatric seizures. I'll page you when he gets here."

Pediatric seizures? That's my first day's introduction to pediatric neurology? I know nothing about seizures! I thought to myself as I headed to the hospital's library. Smartphones and apps were not available yet, so researching in real textbooks and medical journals was my best option.

In the library, I learned that seizures, whether pediatric or adult, are a complex problem of the brain with numerous types of seizures, a plethora of causes, and sometimes-effective treatments. Finding an exact cause or appropriate treatment can be elusive for even the best medical detective. Without seeing my patient first, I was thrown into a trove of medical information, without the ability to narrow down the focus until I could meet and examine my charge.

Childhood seizures are episodes of abnormal electrical activity in the brain that can cause changes in behavior, movement, or consciousness. Pediatric seizures affect around 1/100 children and can present with widely different symptoms.

The cause, severity, and treatment of seizures are highly individualized to each patient's exact problem, if you are lucky enough to find the reason for the seizures. Febrile seizures, or seizures that occur in children with a high fever, usually indicate a better outcome. Many diagnoses of childhood seizures never elucidate a cause, and occasionally, children will "grow out" of their seizure disorder on their own.

After a couple of hours studying in the library, my beeper sounded its alarm, and I dutifully walked back to the ward to meet Dr. Maverick. "Hi Liz, did you learn everything you need to know about pediatric seizures?" he asked with a poker face. I couldn't tell if he was serious or joking.

"I guess we will find out," I replied with a smile. I certainly couldn't let *him* know that I had no idea how to start this investigation into this vexing medical problem in a child.

"Richie is in room #321 with his parents. I'll give you time alone with them. Please come and see me after you have taken a good history and completed your physical exam," he finished.

I had taken copious notes in the library, which I now kept with me on a clipboard. I grabbed my white coat, stethoscope, and notes, and entered Richie's room.

I knocked gently on the door as I stepped into the room and surveyed the scene. The room was filled with sunlight from the floor-to-ceiling window, and Richie was sleeping in the bed. His parents were flanking him. Dad sat on a chair, and Mom sat on the bed, running her fingers through Richie's hair. Both parents were well-dressed and appeared very attentive to their son.

I introduced myself as the student doctor and pulled up a chair at the base of the bed. Many in medicine have likened pediatrics to veterinary medicine, because many times, your patients can't speak for themselves, like a pet or animal. Oftentimes in pediatrics, the parents or guardians are the only historians, as was the case in this situation.

Regardless of whether Richie was asleep or awake, my work on his care would be based on information from his parents. But as luck would have it, these parents were not very good historians, and often, the information I gleaned from them conflicted, depending on who was answering my questions, mom or dad. It made for a confusing interview regarding a confusing illness, but that didn't deter me.

I learned that Richie's mother had had a normal pregnancy without complications. Richie was born by C-section at 40 weeks and had a normal infancy. He had received all of the recommended childhood vaccinations. At age three, things began to change. Richie's mother, who stayed at home with him, began to notice him staring off into space, difficult to arouse from what she called a "trance."

These episodes became more frequent and worrisome. His mom took Richie to his pediatrician, who referred them promptly to a community pediatric neurologist. This physician had diagnosed Richie with "absence seizures" and had started him on medication. Over the preceding year, the community specialist had tried multiple medications for what became worsening seizures. Richie began to exhibit signs of tonic-clonic seizures, denoting a progression of his disease. Finally, he was referred to our big-city, academic institution for further inpatient evaluation.

Richie was admitted to the hospital on three anti-convulsive medicines that were no longer fully controlling his symptoms. But he was so drugged from the heavily sedating meds that he rarely spent time awake, a difficult but not uncommon conundrum. And he was no longer interested in normal childhood activities, such as playing outside or watching television. I couldn't interview him, so I relied exclusively on the report from his parents and the copious records from his two community physicians.

After completing my interview and a physical exam, I left Richie's room and went back to the closet with a computer. I began to sort out my notes from the library, the scribbles from my parents' interview, and the chart notes from the previous outpatient physicians. As if on cue, Dr.

Maverick entered the room and sat next to me. "Well, detective, what do you think is going on?" he asked me straight away.

"To be honest, Dr. Maverick, I feel like this kid is between a rock and a hard place," using a metaphor I hoped would land well. "It seems he has been getting appropriate care in the community; his workup thus far has not been illuminating, but his triple-drug regimen is no longer working, and his symptoms are not improving. He really can't live a normal child's life at this point," I finished.

"What do you think we should do?" he asked me, as though I had any clue about what to do with this precious child.

"Well, he is on three heavily sedating medications that render him into a relatively non-responsive, sleepy state, and he is still having breakthrough symptoms. I wonder what would happen if we stopped all of the medicines and started fresh?" I offered, not knowing if what I had just said was medically legitimate or snake oil.

"Exactly, Liz, good job," Dr. Maverick replied. "It is time for Richie to have a 'drug holiday.' Always remember, first do no harm. Once the drugs have flushed his system, we will have a better picture of his current baseline. It should take about three days. Then, I have a plan for him. Bet you can't guess what my treatment plan is," he stated as he shot me a grin and left the room.

I had no idea what the ultimate plan for Richie was, and I had several days to wait. Each day off the medications, Richie became more alert and interactive with the care team and me. He was an absolutely delightful child with a terrible affliction. His absence seizures returned, but Dr. Maverick elected not to give Richie any traditional medicines. He was saving his "rabbit in the hat" treatment until Richie's system was clear of all prior drugs. Given that Richie had been put on every pediatric seizure drug available at one point or another, I wondered what his plan was.

I didn't have to wait long after Richie's system was clear of the drugs to learn of the new plan. Dr. Maverick was a creative thinker - a rarity for a physician - and he had devised a treatment plan for Richie that would require the approval of the hospital's *ethics* committee. This only served to make me more curious about the plan.

One morning at our usual 7 a.m. meeting, Dr. Maverick let me know that his treatment plan for Richie had been approved by the ethics committee. He shared with me that the plan was unusual, unconventional, and unproven. But the plan may hold the answer for relieving Richie from his life-altering seizures. As we finished our morning meeting with the team, he pulled a quart of extra virgin olive oil from his briefcase and handed it to me, presenting it as a medicine, not a food.

"What on earth do you want me to do with this?" I implored, completely confused. I knew Dr. Maverick had the reputation of being a little "out there," but this seemed *really* out there.

"Have you heard of the 'ketogenic diet', Liz?" he asked.

"Yes, of course. Atkins. That kind of diet?" I replied.

"Yes, but the treatment we are going to try on Richie is a diet consisting 100% of olive oil. No food or any drinks, except water," he continued. "Ketones, from a ketogenic diet, are the preferred fuel for the brain. I hypothesize that we can stem his seizures with a strict, ketogenic diet."

"Fascinating. With all due respect, sir, how do you plan to get a four-year-old to drink olive oil?" I asked sincerely.

"We will place a nasogastric (NG) tube if needed. He will need 1½ cups of extra virgin olive oil per day, divided into three doses of ½ cup at each feeding. We should have results in a week or so after he is in ketosis. Please discuss the plan with his parents," he finished.

It was at times like these that I felt completely inept in medicine, despite my nearly five years of learning. I felt incapable of both describing a treatment plan and getting the parents' buy-in and consent for a regimen that I did not fully grasp myself. And at that time, there was literally no information in textbooks or medical journals about this unconventional treatment plan.

I entered Richie's room and was pleasantly surprised that both parents were there. After a thorough explanation of the plan for Richie, both parents eagerly agreed to try the ketogenic diet consisting 100% of olive oil. They truly felt they had exhausted all other options, as did Dr. Maverick and I.

Even though Richie was pretty alert after his drug holiday, there was still no way we were going to get him to drink olive oil. An NG tube was placed, and the unconventional treatment was administered directly into his stomach. Fortunately, the oil filled him up, so he wasn't hungry or begging for food. Richie spent a couple of weeks in the hospital on the ketogenic diet and off all of the medicines he had been on at the time of admission. He did not have any more seizures while an inpatient: The experiment had worked. Spectacularly.

Richie's parents were exceptionally grateful for his care and unconventional treatment plan. They saw Dr. Maverick as a hero, as I did. Richie was discharged on a modified ketogenic diet, and to the best of my knowledge, he did not have another seizure.

Chapter 14
Skinny Girl

Toward the end of my clinical rotations in medical school, I was assigned to a stint in the university hospital on the internal medicine service. It had the reputation of being an extremely busy rotation with overnight call at the hospital every 72 hours. Although I knew I had a horrendous month ahead of me with significant time away from my family, I was buoyed by the knowledge that medical school was nearing its end.

On my first day on the service, I joined the large team of medical students, interns, residents, and attending physicians in the doctor's lounge. I was the only woman on the service except for our boss. The attending physician, Dr. Youthful, was a serious-looking, middle-aged woman who gave us the impression that she still had something to prove. She let us all know this month was going to be "brutal" with regards to our patient load and complexity.

It took all my nerve not to roll my eyes. I was so exhausted from five years of medical school and the birth and growth of my young family. I was becoming jaded at the thought of working more 100-hour work weeks as a medical student.

Per usual, the large census of patients was divided up among the team. Dr. Youthful turned toward me, the only other female in the room, and said, "Liz, I want you to take the patient in room #369. She has been in the hospital for a week or so, and she does not do well with male providers. She is admitted for life-threatening anorexia nervosa, but is actually getting worse by the day here. She may need medical intervention soon."

I, of course, had heard of anorexia nervosa, but had not worked with a hospitalized patient with this diagnosis before. Once the team had dispersed with their assignments, I headed to the library to do a little research before seeing my patient. There, I learned a lot about the subject.

Anorexia affects young women most commonly and manifests with an intense fear of gaining weight and a distorted body image. Anorexics also exhibit extreme behavior around food, which includes restrictive eating, excessive exercise, and sometimes purging. I had seen many people over my lifetime who would likely qualify as anorexic, but had never worked with someone so afflicted with the disease that they required hospitalization.

Anorexia is caused by a combination of genetic predisposition, psychological factors, environmental influences, and most importantly, the patient's desire for control in their life. Sometimes, the intake of food into their body is all they feel they have left in life to influence. I also learned that anorexia nervosa has one of the highest mortality rates of all psychological afflictions at 25%. The leading cause of mortality in anorexics is heart failure.

While many may consider anorexia to be a volitional, vanity disease, I approached my new patient with detached neutrality. I found a study in the library that likened anorexics to prisoners of WWII, who were starved by their captors. The lack of a reliable food source - like in war - elucidates the same behavior as anorexics: food hoarding, food elimination, incessant playing with their food, and fear of eating.

It appeared from my research that one's food behavior can be influenced by psychological factors both in and out of one's control. My patient was hospitalized when her mother said she would not let her daughter attend college unless she "got cured" of her anorexia. I was excited to meet her and hoped I could help in some way.

My new patient's name was Krystal. She was placed on a medical floor, rather than the psychiatric ward, due to her unstable and life-threatening chemistries. She had already been hospitalized for a week before I met her, so I took the opportunity to read her entire chart before introducing myself. I grabbed her paper chart from its cubby outside her room and found an available computer at the nearest nurses' station.

In reading her chart, I learned that Krystal had refused most meals and all medications over the preceding week while hospitalized. She appeared to not like men and had refused to work with several of my male colleagues. She had insisted on weighing herself several times a day until the nurses took the scale out of her room, making her very angry. She was generally irritable and non-compliant, becoming difficult for the staff to manage. I hoped that as a woman, I might be able to make an inroad with her.

Upon admission, Krystal had refused all interventions, such as an IV with electrolytes or any oral sustenance. In the week before meeting her, she had had a cardiac echocardiogram, which showed she had severe heart failure due to her illness, putting her life in great danger. She seemed to have no desire to get better, and our attempts to help her had been met with indifference or contempt.

I walked the halls of the hospital until I found room #369. Krystal was 17 years old, 5' 3", and weighed 80 pounds upon admission to our hospital. Her BMI was 14, which was very low. The morning I saw her, she had weighed in at 81 pounds, which displeased her immensely. This left her in a particularly foul mood. I walked into Krystal's room and gasped quietly under my breath. The girl in the bed before me looked like a concentration camp survivor. She looked diminutive, unhappy, and tired.

"Hi, Krystal, I'm Liz, the student doctor who will be taking care of you," I offered as I sat down on a chair next to her bed. "Would it be okay if I asked you a few questions?"

"If you have to," Krystal replied in an irritated tone as she looked out the window and away from me.

"Why don't we start by talking about your family, and your role in it." I started. I hoped that if we took the magnifying glass off of her, she might be more forthcoming.

"What do you want to know? My family sucks," she offered.

"Why don't you tell me what *you* want me to know?" I replied. What ensued after that was a 60-minute conversation, giving me a lot of information about her life. She seemed to warm up to me and appeared to relax a bit. I felt hopeful at that moment.

Krystal reported she came from a wealthy family where appearances were "everything," including maintaining a slim physique. She had had a very negative interaction with her father at age 11, which started her desire to be in total control of her life. Her father had publicly humiliated her at a family reunion by calling her "pudgy" and "fat," a verboten body habitus in her family, setting off her journey with anorexia.

It became apparent that after the family shaming, Krystal felt the only thing that she could control in her life was the food she would, or wouldn't, put into her mouth. A silent rebellion starting at age 11 that had set her off on an illness that had consumed the totality of her teenage years up to that point.

After the public humiliation by her father regarding her appearance, Krystal began to change her lifestyle and eating habits. She expressed intense fear of weight gain and a distorted body image - and now she believed she was still fat at 81 pounds. She also reported extreme behaviors, including excessive exercise, severely restrictive eating habits, and purging (a very bad sign). Her disease had progressed year after year, and she had very poor self-esteem.

I performed a brief physical examination on Krystal, which she reluctantly agreed to. While she was most likely an attractive person at one point, her emaciated appearance and sparse hair on her head made her look almost elderly. Her skin was pale gray and cold to the touch, and her heart rate was slow and faint. Her fingernails were split and peeling off her fingers, and her limbs were like twigs. I had never seen so many malnourished bones protruding on a live body. It was sad for me to see her in such a state.

Krystal exhibited signs of perfectionism and would frequently pick invisible lint off her hospital gown as we spoke. She also tugged at her hair incessantly, pulling out strand after strand and placing the hair in a pile on her lap. She reported fatigue, poor sleep, and an obsession with her appearance. She had seen a couple of therapists over the years, but no one had been able to make inroads with her.

Krystal had been told by Dr. Youthful that if she didn't start to gain weight, she had a high likelihood of dying. Unfortunately, due to the late stage of her disease, she let Krystal know that nutrition might not save her life and could actually hasten her death due to "refeeding syndrome." This is a potentially life-threatening condition that can occur when nutrition is reintroduced too quickly after a long period of starvation.

Refeeding syndrome causes rapid shifts in electrolytes, such as potassium and magnesium, which can lead to serious complications like heart failure and death. This information, when relayed to Krystal, had started a rift between Dr. Youthful and her. Krystal felt that this information endorsed her desire *not* to eat. She argued that if eating could kill her, then she shouldn't eat. No solution for Krystal was easy or ideal, and she was very manipulative with the medical team.

I reiterated Dr. Youthful's concerns and asked Krystal if she had any plans to start eating. She said she had ordered lunch for the first time since admission, and promised me that she would eat something. I let her know that if she didn't start eating, the next step would be to place a nasogastric (NG) tube for feeding her, which she let me know she would decline. She told me that she had lost the desire to go to college, so she didn't see the need for any anorexia intervention or reason to please her mother.

I eventually left Krystal's room and searched for Dr. Youthful. I found her outside of another patient's room.

"Hi, Dr. Youthful, I have finished my time with Krystal," I reported.

"What do you think, Liz?" she replied.

"I think she's in trouble. Her echocardiogram shows an ejection fraction of only 30%, indicating end-stage cardiac illness," I offered. "She has no desire to get well, it seems. I discussed an NG tube with her, but she refused."

"Did you see her potassium level?" Dr. Youthful asked.

"Yes, 2.4, another bad sign," I replied. Extremely low potassium, a common occurrence with anorexia, can cause sudden cardiac death.

"Well, she's been here for a week, declining *any* interventions, and seemingly getting worse. What do you think we should do?" she asked.

"To my surprise, she agreed to eat lunch today. I will plan to see her around that time and report back to you," I finished.

"Good job, Liz. That is great to hear," Dr. Sincere replied. "But while that may sound good right now, you have to take everything an anorexic promises with a grain of salt. They will often lie to appease the current situation," Dr. Youthful finished. I felt that her cynicism seemed a bit harsh, but I had to admit to myself that I had no experience working with anorexics.

I went back to Krystal's room after lunch was served. True to form, Krystal had ordered a low-fat, vegan meal. I entered the room and observed the culinary mayhem. She had picked apart the entire tray of food and arranged the food in an exact pattern of her initials on her tray. Tiny pieces of tofu, bits of cooked carrots, and a green salad were rendered relatively unidentifiable. It was impossible to tell if she had eaten a single bite, but I assumed her empty mouth was a good indicator that she had not eaten anything.

"Can you remove this tray?" Krystal asked as soon as I entered the room. "It's really stressing me out."

I complied and removed the tray. "Krystal, did you eat anything?" I asked earnestly.

"I couldn't. I just don't want anything in my mouth," she replied. "And this food is disgusting!" That was a sentiment I couldn't disagree with. Hospitals are generally not known for their cuisine.

"How about we order you a milkshake?" I asked, hoping it would appeal.

"Whatever," she relented. "Chocolate."

Even though Krystal had indeed lied about her intention to eat lunch, I was elated at the idea that I had made a culinary inroad with her. I went and grabbed a chocolate milkshake from the cafeteria, paid for it with my own money, and brought it back to Krystal. She promised she would drink it. As I had other patients to attend to and didn't want her to feel pressured to drink the shake in front of me, I left her alone with the milkshake.

I came back to Krystal's room a couple of hours later and found her throwing up in the bathroom, ridding herself of any milkshake calories. I left the room before she saw me, very discouraged. I then found her nurse and placed an order to have her bathroom door locked. Her latest antics had earned her a revocation of bathroom privileges.

I went back to Krystal's room a couple of hours later, before I left the hospital for the evening. Krystal was resting and listening to music on her CD player. I pulled up a chair next to her bed and decided to have a straight-talk conversation with her myself, something I hadn't done yet.

"Krystal, I tried to visit you earlier today when you were throwing up your milkshake," I stated bluntly. I was starting to feel discouraged with her situation myself, and it left me feeling impotent. "We need to have a serious conversation now," I continued. "You are in a very precarious situation. Your potassium level and heart failure put you at great risk of dying."

"Why does everyone here want me to *live* so badly?" Krystal asked in reply. "Why can't you just leave me alone?"

"To be honest, Krystal, what we want for you is pretty immaterial at this point. What is important is what do *you* want for your future?" I asked.

"I just want to be left alone," she reiterated. "I'm tired of everyone telling me I'm too skinny. I don't know why you all can't see how fat I am," she replied. I knew enough by that point in the rotation that any verbal attempt to get Krystal to see herself through another lens was futile and would likely only alienate her further. I realized our conversation was essentially over, and I had little to offer at that point. I decided, with a discouraged resignation, to go home.

Over the ensuing week, the decision was made by Dr. Youthful to discharge Krystal in the near future if she continued to decline any intervention or treatment. She indicated that due to her age and competency, there was nothing we could do to force Krystal to accept an NG tube or other life-saving interventions. I let Krystal know the plan to discharge her, which she accepted with the same disengaged resignation she exhibited around food. Complete indifference. It was hard to tell if Krystal truly understood the danger she was in.

A couple of days later, I arrived at the hospital early as usual to pre-round on my patients before the team meeting at 7 a.m. I logged on to the computer to "pull my list" of patients. Only this morning, Krystal was missing from my list. I was surprised and puzzled. *Had she been transferred to the psychiatric ward? Did Dr. Youthful discharge her without telling me?* I wondered. It didn't take long before the mystery was solved.

After the room had filled up with the group for our morning meeting, Dr. Youthful arrived a few minutes late. "Well, team, we had a death overnight," Dr. Youthful reported. "Our end-stage anorexic, Krystal, succumbed to her disease last night. Cause of death: heart failure." She looked at me and said, "I'm sorry, Liz, I know you tried."

Although I knew that Krystal's death was certainly a possible outcome, it was shocking to think that her life was taken at such a young age. I hoped and prayed that she had finally found peace and nutrition on the other side.

Chapter 15
Gut Feeling

In my fifth and final year of medical school, I was assigned to a month at a community infectious disease clinic. My boss, Dr. Infection, was a nationally known and highly regarded physician in the community and the country. His name was on all of the relevant infectious disease textbooks and journal articles, denoting mastery of the specialty. His reputation was one of a combination of high intellect and an envious bedside manner. Given that infectious diseases are one of the most common causes of doctor visits, hospital admissions, and death, I was excited to learn from him.

Unlike all of the other physicians I had worked with up to that date, Dr. Infection emailed me personally before the rotation began. He expressed his interest in my upcoming time with him and invited me to join him on the first morning of the rotation at the adjacent hospital's Doctor's

Dining Room (DDR). I was impressed with his unorthodox and welcoming approach to my next month of learning.

I arrived on my first day at 7 a.m. and took a seat in the DDR after pouring myself a cup of coffee. A few minutes later, Dr. Infection breezed into the room with a happy smile on his face. After working with so many burnt-out and unpleasant physicians, I was hopeful this rotation would be different.

Dr. Infection took a seat next to me and introduced himself. "Hi, you must be Liz. I'm Dr. Infection. So glad to meet you. Welcome to infectious disease!"

Dr. Infection asked me lots of questions about myself, and upon learning that I had two young children at home, he let me know that he would "go easy" on me during our time together. He even promised I would be home by dinnertime on most days, a first for me in medical school. He indicated that his infectious disease practice was more of a "boutique" practice with a gentle cadence to his day. "Now, I'm not saying this month will be easy, but you should be able to learn what you need to know for your board exam without sacrificing your family time," he offered. I was thrilled with what I was hearing.

Dr. Infection would often see patients whose diagnosis had evaded other physicians. He was considered the "last resort," or final detective, for vexing infectious disease cases or other medical illnesses with an unknown origin. The mix of patients and their accompanying unusual medical diagnoses made for an interesting month. I spent hours reviewing blood work and cultures under a microscope, and learned the appropriate antibiotic, antiviral, antifungal, or antiparasitic to address each "bug." I got the feeling that I wouldn't be seeing a simple garden variety of infectious diseases during my month, and I was right.

One day, early in my rotation with Dr. Infection, he let me know we were going to see an "interesting" patient that morning. I had learned over and over in my stint as a medical student that you never want to be an "interesting case" to a doctor, as it usually indicates a mystery yet to be solved or some kind of bad diagnosis.

"Liz, we have a patient named Jessica coming in this morning. I'd like you to see her first, then come and find me and let me know your thoughts on her diagnosis," Dr. Infection stated. "She has seen two doctors already for her weight loss, but her diagnosis has remained elusive."

"No problem," I replied. "Are there any notes to review first?" I asked.

"Yes, all of the records from her previous physician visits are in her chart," he replied as he handed me a thick, new patient chart to review.

I had over an hour before Jessica's appointment and took the opportunity to comb through her extensive chart. She had seen her primary care physician (PCP) numerous times and even a psychiatrist. No one to date had been able to find the cause of her consistent weight loss, causing her PCP to "dump her" on the psychiatrist in a fit of medical desperation. A visit to an infectious disease doctor was just another attempt to elucidate a diagnosis for her. I was hopeful Dr. Infection would be able to help her.

"How did the chart review go, Liz?" Dr. Infection asked me before Jessica arrived. "Any brilliant thoughts about what might be going on with her?"

"To be honest, sir, I'm not really sure what to think. The previous physician seems to have been pretty thorough with all of the bloodwork she's had in the last six months. But she was of normal weight to start with, and she's lost 30 pounds in the last six months, unintentionally," I replied. Unintentional weight loss in most patients is a serious cause for concern, and usually indicates something bad, like cancer. "Hopefully, I will be able to find out something new when I see her," I finished.

Jessica arrived and was placed in an exam room by the medical assistant. I entered the room alone and introduced myself. "Hi Jessica, I'm Liz, a student doctor working with Dr. Infection. He has asked me to see you first, and he will see you after you and I are finished. Can you please share with me what's been going on with your weight loss?" I asked.

"I haven't tried to lose weight," Jessica immediately replied. "I eat a lot of food, but I still keep losing weight. I also have pretty bad stomach cramps after I eat. My primary care doctor thinks my weight loss is all in my head! He even sent me to a psychiatrist, but that didn't go well," she said with a sarcastic tone. I could sense her frustration.

Jessica was 30 years old, very attractive, and worked in retail. She lived alone in a nice part of town and was engaged to get married. She was indeed very thin and looked somewhat malnourished to me. I took a thorough history from her, or so I thought, and came up empty-handed for the cause of her weight loss.

I tried to uncover all possible reasons for her losing weight, including anorexia nervosa or bulimia, but nothing rang true. Jessica denied any desire to lose weight at all. I had to admit, I was baffled. I performed a brief physical examination, then I left Jessica in her room and exited it to find Dr. Infection. I found him in his office working on a new chapter for an upcoming textbook publication on infectious diseases. I sat down in a chair in his office.

"Dr. Infection, I am stumped and not really sure Jessica belongs in an infectious disease clinic," I offered. "Maybe we should refer her back to the psychiatrist?" I finished, but immediately regretted what I had said.

Dr. Infection graciously ignored my reference to the psychiatrist and then proceeded to "pimp" me about all the information I had gleaned from my interview with Jessica. He kept asking me for more and more information, seeking to see if I had uncovered anything that the previous physicians had missed. After a few minutes, it appeared that Dr. Infection had tapped my limited knowledge and indicated it was time for him to see her himself. The puzzler was going to go to work now.

"Well, let's go see her together," Dr. Infection replied as he stood up from his desk. "I have a few questions for her that I don't think you asked." I felt a bit sheepish at that moment, but had to admit that he was probably right.

Dr. Infection gently knocked on the exam room door before entering. He introduced himself, and we sat in our respective chairs. "Hi Jessica, I'm Dr. Infection. I have one question for you. Where have you traveled in the past year?" he asked.

His question left me speechless as it was the one question I, and other previous physicians, had failed to ask her. A feeling of incompetence and embarrassment washed over me when I realized this was the exact question I *should* have asked her.

"I have traveled to Mexico a couple of times," Jessica answered.

"Where in Mexico did you stay? A resort?" he asked in reply.

"No, my fiancé and I like to stay with the locals when we travel," she said. "We usually camp on the beach."

Dr. Infection then proceeded to perform a physical exam on Jessica. Her hip and rib bones protruded from her frame, giving an eerie sight. Dr. Infection palpated her concave abdomen and listened for bowel sounds. Once he was finished, he helped Jessica sit back up on the exam table, and sat himself back down on the exam stool in front of her.

"Jessica, I believe I know what is causing your weight loss," he said. I couldn't wait to hear his thoughts, as I still had no clue. "I suspect you have an infection in your colon, most likely from your travel to Mexico. There is a worm found in contaminated foods or water that can get stuck in your body, causing weight loss. Basically, the worm takes over your gut, feeds itself on *your* nourishment, and robs your body of nutrition. I believe I can help you," he continued. "We will need to do a few tests to confirm my suspicion, but once identified, the treatment is not difficult," he finished.

After answering Jessica's questions, Dr. Infection and I excused ourselves from the exam room and reconvened in his office. "Intestinal worm infections can cause a range of symptoms, including abdominal pain, diarrhea, nausea, and weight loss. I'm happy we most likely found her problem. Now comes the fun part, Liz," he said to me as we both sat down.

I was forever grateful that he didn't humiliate me for neglecting to ask the one question that would have been helpful to him. "Now we need to schedule her for a barium swallow to confirm the diagnosis. We do that here in the office. Let's get her scheduled before your time on this rotation ends," he finished. *Note to self: don't forget to ask patients about travel*, I thought to myself.

I decided it was time to learn more about intestinal worm infections, as I had clearly missed the mark with Jessica. I learned four main types that affect humans and animals - roundworms, tapeworms, hookworms, and pinworms. Most worms are contracted through contaminated food, water, or soil. They are found most commonly in less developed countries, such as Mexico, but can arise anywhere.

Symptoms from a worm infection vary from mild to severe, and can ultimately result in weight loss, malnutrition, and organ damage. Prevention includes cooking food thoroughly, proper hygiene, and avoiding contaminated water. I learned that an unaddressed infection from one of these worms can be very serious, as in Jessica's situation.

We saw Jessica a week later for a barium swallow, my first experience with the test. After swallowing the barium drink, a radiopaque liquid that tastes like chalk, we moved her to the clinic's procedure room. We waited for the medicine to flush through her GI system before imaging her abdomen with a fluoroscopic X-ray. The procedure revealed that her intestines were chock-full of a round worm called ascariasis, most likely picked up in Mexico.

During the procedure, Dr. Infection pointed out the numerous, foot-long worms that were now visible in black and white, clogging her colon. It looked like cooked spaghetti inside her body, and it took all my professional might not to gag at that point. He gently gave Jessica the news that her GI tract was filled with these worms, happily robbing her of nutrition.

Dr. Infection then described to her the unpleasant, but necessary, passage of these worms through her system after treatment with the appropriate drug. Seeing these worms in the toilet bowl can be an unnerving experience, and Dr. Infection wanted her to be prepared.

Once back in his office, Dr. Infection said, "Liz, if this infection had continued much longer, Jessica could have had a complete bowel obstruction from these buggers, risking her life. It's awesome that we saw her before this issue got any worse." He continued, "the treatment from here is pretty straightforward, and she should have a good outcome." I couldn't believe he kept referring to "we" as I had contributed next to nothing to the case. His words were an endearing nod to our upcoming collegiality once I graduated from school. It was also a nod to Dr. Infection's overall kindness.

Jessica was given the appropriate medicine for roundworms and was expected to recover completely. As I had my own trip to Mexico planned in the near future after that rotation, I gratefully allowed Dr. Infection to provide me with the appropriate medications to keep my own GI tract safe. He really was a gentleman physician, with an excellent bedside manner, and my time with him was one of the best in medical school.

Chapter 16
Danger in the OR

Of all the medical specialties, surgical programs are usually considered the most competitive: Neurosurgery, orthopedic surgery, transplant surgery, plastic surgery, and so on. The surgical residencies are among the longest and most difficult of all specialties, and admittance to a program is highly competitive. Even if you are at the top of your medical school class, you still may not match in a surgical specialty.

Usually, in addition to four years of medical school, if you want to specialize in surgery, you must also take an additional year consisting of research in your desired surgical field, or take a year in the pathology department. Only the top students, and lucky ones at that, match in surgical specialties.

In my fifth and last year of medical school, I was assigned to the general surgery service at our university's hospital. It was known for being a very difficult service, requiring 100-hour work weeks and overnight call at the hospital every 72 hours. As a student, you would be primarily responsible for seeing patients on the service both before and after surgery, managing their care *outside* of the OR. Getting invited into the OR as a student on this service was a rare and coveted activity.

The general surgery service varies greatly depending on where you are located geographically in the United States. Cities and large towns will have many surgical subspecialties, while small towns may only have general surgeons, who perform a wider variety of operations.

In the city where I was attending school, all of the surgical specialties were represented, leaving the general surgery service to attend to a "garden variety" of general surgical problems, such as hernia repairs, cancer removal, and gall bladder removal. Occasionally, we would see an oddball diagnosis, and even more occasionally, a student would be invited to join the senior team in the OR for the patient's surgery.

On my first day in my tenure on the month-long service, the team met at 6 a.m. in the surgical office to plan for the day's activities. The chief of our service, Dr. Sincere, was a middle-aged woman whose reputation preceded her. She was known as being exceptionally demanding of the team on her service, but also known as being exceedingly kind and encouraging, almost "motherly." She was the only female head of a surgical department at our institution, and I was excited to work with her.

The surgical team I was assigned to consisted of the chief, three male surgical residents, two male medical students, and me. Per usual, we all sat in a cramped room and introduced ourselves to each other. By this time in my medical school tenure, I was used to being the lone woman on the team, and these surgeons really intimidated me. I was grateful for Dr. Sincere, and I looked forward to learning from her.

As I was the only other female on the service with Dr. Sincere, she took me under her wing and gave me unconditional support. Dr. Sincere was surprised to learn that I had had two children while in medical school. She let me know that she had given up on the dream of being a mother when she chose to be a general surgeon and work in academia. I got the impression that she was a bit wistful about that decision. She did let me know that this month-long rotation would be very demanding for a young mother - no special treatment for me. I braced myself for another long month away from my husband and children.

Over my first week on the service, I spent quite a bit of time with Dr. Sincere outside of the OR at her pre- and post-op patients' bedside. I found the general surgery service to be an offshoot of the cadaver lab. I was glad I remembered so much detailed anatomy from my time there, four years earlier. I quickly found out that as a general surgeon, intimate knowledge of the human body was essential both inside and outside the OR. Dr. Sincere "pimped me" mercilessly on anatomy, and I did my best to answer her queries correctly.

As Dr. Sincere's protege, she allowed me to do a lot of minor procedures outside of the operating room as I accompanied her to visit her patients on the wards. Dressing changes, tube and drain removal, suture removal, and more. She seemed to be pleased with my performance and indicated she would allow me to join her in the OR before the rotation was over. This only served to make me work harder and put in even longer hours, missing precious time with my family. It became clear pretty quickly that surgery demands so much from those who pursue the specialty.

In the second week of my surgical rotation, Dr. Sincere approached me after our usual morning meeting and once we were alone in the office. "Liz, you have impressed me this past week. You seem to have a knack for anatomy and surgery. Would you like to join me in the OR soon?"

"I would love to, Dr. Sincere," I answered, flattered at the invitation. To my knowledge, I was the only medical student thus far on this rotation who had received such an invitation from her. I hoped it wouldn't bring out the jealousy of my male comrades.

"Great, let me look at the upcoming surgeries this week, and I'll find a good one for you to hold the retractor," she shot back with a smile as she left the office and headed to the operating room.

Yay! More retractor holding, I thought sarcastically as I left the office myself and got to work on the wards with the post-op patients.

Later that day, I ran into Dr. Sincere as she was exiting the OR after a particularly brutal operation. "Sometimes I seriously wonder *why* I chose this specialty, Liz," she confessed to me. "I would love to tell you to become a surgeon, but I don't know any longer if I could do that in good conscience. I've just finished what was supposed to be a simple gall bladder removal, but it turned into a nightmare due to adhesions from a previous surgery. The laparoscopic procedure turned into an open surgical disaster and completely derailed my day. Thank goodness the patient survived. Please follow him on the wards; he is in room #808."

"No problem, Dr. Sincere, I've got him covered," I replied.

The next morning at our usual 6 a.m. meeting, Dr. Sincere addressed me directly in front of the group. "Liz, there is a new admission I would like you to pick up. He's in the emergency department right now and will be coming up to the wards soon. He will most likely need surgery," she continued. "Please get him tucked in and page me when you are done with your physical exam and assessment."

Dr. Sincere had not divulged the new patient's diagnosis, so I had little to go on to know how to proceed. I checked his ER labs and notes on the computer. It seemed that our new patient was being admitted for an infection in his lower legs. He was initially diagnosed with cellulitis in the ER, a bacterial infection that can progress rapidly and can even result in death if left unchecked. I readied myself to meet him by doing a little computer research on cellulitis while I waited for him to arrive on the ward.

I met my new patient, Eddie, after the orderlies settled him in in his room. I let him rest for a minute, then I entered the room and introduced myself. "Hi, Eddie, I'm Liz, a student doctor who will be following you while you are in the hospital."

Eddie was 30 years old and an IV drug user. He looked much older than his age. He appeared to be in a *lot* of pain, despite the morphine drip he had been put on in the ER. He was clearly in a very bad mood, and my presence did nothing to comfort him.

"A *student doctor*? How did I get so lucky?" Eddie asked sarcastically as he rolled his eyes. "Will I actually get to see a *real doctor*?"

"Yes, Eddie, you will have a team of real doctors that will follow you while you are here. I am just the low person on the doctor totem pole," I confessed in an attempt to diffuse the situation. "You are in good hands with our group," I replied, trying to impart confidence in my participation in his care. I was reassured that no matter what Eddie thought of me, Dr. Sincere would not take me off his case. Instead, if necessary, she would lecture him about the benefits of a "teaching hospital" and put him in his place.

I took a detailed history from Eddie before I performed a physical exam on him. When I met him, his body was covered by the bed sheet. Eddie admitted to being an IV drug user for over a decade. Despite his habits - and preference for IV heroin - he had had very few complications or problems arising from his drug use over his lifetime. He was employed in construction and lived on his own, independently in an apartment in a bad part of town.

As is common with IV drug use, Eddie had started to "blow out" his veins from repeated use of the toxins and contaminants associated with IV drugs. As a solution to his diminishing veins to inject, Eddie had begun to "skin pop" his drug of choice into his lower legs. He chose his legs as he was able to cover his tracks with the blue jeans he wore for work. Recently, his legs had begun to swell and cause great discomfort. So painful that he had to cut back on his drug use. I surmised his bad mood could also be a result of withdrawal symptoms, as well as the infection. He certainly didn't look like he felt well at all.

I performed a physical exam on Eddie as much as I could without pulling back the sheet to reveal his legs. He was slender and had tracks on his arms that emerged from the too-big hospital gown. He was relatively uncooperative and unpleasant, but he ultimately allowed me to do my job.

"Okay, Eddie, it's time to examine your legs," I said toward the end of our exam.

"Do your thing," he shot back as he threw off the sheet, revealing his problem.

Oh my God, you have got to be kidding me, this is bad, really bad! I thought to myself as I viewed his calves. "Eddie, how long have your legs been so red and swollen?" I asked.

"Well, about a month. I've continued to use drugs," he replied honestly.

The man lying before me looked relatively normal from the knees up, but his calves belied the problem in full view. Eddie's calves were deep red and swollen to double their size, nearly approximating the circumference of his thighs.

His skin was hot and painful to the touch, with 2+ pitting edema. Several open areas on each calf were weeping green-colored pus that smelled terrible. I started to hold my breath as I finished the exam.

I took a Sharpie out of my coat pocket and drew a "margin line" at the top of Eddie's calves where the redness stopped. This is a low-tech way to watch and see if the cellulitis has progressed over time. I used the pen to outline the top red margin just below his knees. I also wrote the date and time on his thigh of my assessment of his current condition.

This Sharpie demarcation would be monitored closely by the team and me, and would be used as a signal that Eddie's condition was improving or worsening. Advancing cellulitis can be deadly, and quickly so. I wrote an order for the nursing staff to monitor the line of demarcation every hour and to call me with any changes.

I wrote Eddie's admission orders and covered him with broad-spectrum antibiotics to cover the most common causes of cellulitis in an IV drug user. I also made sure he would have the appropriate dose of pain medication. Pain control in addicts can be very difficult because their tolerance to opioids is so high.

Many physicians don't address this issue at all, and chronically underdose pain medicine for addicts, oftentimes due to judgment about their drug habit. Despite his foul mood and irreverent treatment of me, I ordered him the appropriate - and *very* high dose of morphine - to make him comfortable.

A couple of hours later, I received a page from Dr. Sincere. While I had been attending to other patients, she had gone and seen Eddie herself. I called her back immediately.

"Liz, we've got an emergency here," she stated. "I just saw Eddie and read your good admission note. His cellulitis has already advanced a centimeter since you made your mark a few hours ago. We've got to get him into the OR immediately and release the pressure on his calves, or he is headed toward bilateral amputation. I'd like you to join me today. Meet me in OR #6 in an hour."

I was surprised and thrilled with the offer. Per usual, I stuffed a little food in my mouth and took a bathroom break before heading to the OR. Once there, I met Dr. Sincere at the scrub sink.

"What do you think is going on, Liz?" Dr. Sincere asked me as she scrubbed in.

"Well, he certainly has really bad cellulitis," I replied as I began to suds up my own hands and arms.

"Actually, Eddie's problem has progressed way beyond cellulitis at this point. He now has bilateral necrotizing fasciitis, a life-threatening condition," she offered. "This is going to be a bloody, purulent mess. Brace yourself."

"Necrotizing fasciitis? This should be interesting! I thought to myself, having only learned about this problem in textbooks.

We entered the OR together and donned our sterile garb with the help of the scrub nurse. Eddie was already on the table and anesthetized. The nurses had prepped his legs for surgery, and Dr. Sincere and I took our places at the end of the bed and got ready to go to work. I was immediately handed a retractor.

Dr. Sincere talked me through the procedure and gave me a lot of information about the disease we were seeing. Necrotizing fasciitis is also known as a flesh-eating condition. It occurs when an infection is found in an enclosed space in the body, often between muscle bundles, as in Eddie's case. Unbeknownst to him, the lower leg is one of the worst places to inject drugs, as the calf has three separate compartments of various muscles in a relatively small space.

The infection, caused by dirty needles and bad drugs, gets trapped in a tight muscle bundle and begins to swell, often under great pressure. If the infection spreads, this can cause a rapid decline in the patient's blood supply to his muscles that could result in amputation or even death.

The goal of the surgery was to simply relieve the pressure on Eddie's calf muscles, hoping to avoid a double amputation. "Simple", however, is a misnomer. I watched as Dr. Sincere cut multiple full-length, vertical incisions deep into his calves and into the fascia in an attempt to relieve the pressure on the muscles. As she cut Eddie's flesh, pus and blood extruded from both legs, which I helped to clean up as best I could. The smell of the pus was foul, indicating an infection, and my mask did little to protect me from the odor. I held the retractor, tried not to gag, and agreed it certainly was a bloody, infected mess.

Dr. Sincere then asked the head OR nurse to hand her an intracompartmental pressure measurement device (ICP). She inserted the catheter into various muscle bundles in Eddie's lower legs. Each time she read a pressure reading, she let out a groan of frustration. She shouted numbers out to the room and seemed to get more agitated by the minute. "33! 42! 55!" She handed the device back to the head OR nurse and addressed me directly.

"Liz, I am not getting the result I need to save his legs. The pressure on his muscles is still too high. Any pressure over 30 mmHg can be deadly. I'm going to have to change tactics here," Dr. Sincere admitted.

Looking at Eddie's infected muscles dissected and splayed out before me, I had no idea what she could be talking about. *What else can she possibly do, except amputate? I* wondered. At this point, Dr. Sincere took her gloved hand and placed it into Eddie's right calf. She dug her fingers in between two muscle bundles and ran her hand up and down the calf in an attempt to relieve some pressure and to extrude more pus.

"Oh my God! Ouch! What the hell?" Dr. Sincere shouted excitedly, startling the whole team in the operating room.

"Are you okay?" I asked reflexively, not understanding what had just happened.

"No! This motherf***er has needles buried in his muscles!" she replied as she pulled her hand away from his body. "I just got stuck by a couple of needles!" I learned this can happen when addicts reuse syringes to the point that the needle comes apart from the syringe and remains lodged in the body. It now appeared that Eddie had innumerable needle fragments housed within his infected legs.

Dr. Sincere immediately took off her breached glove and went to a sink in the OR to wash away the blood on her fingers. While still at the sink, attempting to scrub out the patient's blood from hers, she addressed the head scrub nurse, "Susie, do we have this patient's HIV and Hep C status?"

"No, Dr. Sincere. We don't," Susie replied.

"Please order an HIV and Hepatitis panel, STAT," she replied.

Dr. Sincere replaced her gloves with a new, sterile set and returned to the operating table. "Liz, Eddie has needle fragments buried in his muscles, so we can't do any more work here. Anytime there is an infection with pus, like here, we can't close up his wounds with sutures. You can never leave 'pus under pressure.' We will have to leave his leg wounds open for now."

Eddie left the OR with his legs looking like they had gone through a meat grinder. We finished the case, and Dr. Sincere educated me about how to handle a needle stick. Both she and Eddie would follow a predetermined protocol, and they would both be immediately tested for HIV. Depending on the results, more or less testing over the next three months would be required.

Eddie's HIV results came back as positive, heightening the fear and anxiety of the needle stick for Dr. Sincere. Fortunately, I found out later that Dr. Sincere never tested positive for HIV or hepatitis.

I followed Eddie for a couple of days after his surgery, but in the end, there was no way to turn back time. He succumbed to his infection before amputation was ever considered.

Interlogue
Introduction to Internship & Residency

Medical School, unless you attend Harvard, is defined by the wearing of a short, white coat, making you easy to identify in the clinic or on the hospital wards. The longer white coat is reserved for interns, residents, and full-fledged doctors. Graduation from medical school is marked by purchasing and embossing your name onto a full-length lab coat. A rite of passage.

"Liz Casper, M.D." was embroidered on my left side above my breast pocket. As a graduation gift from my family, I was given a "doctor's bag" filled with a blood pressure cuff, a new stethoscope, an otoscope, an ophthalmoscope, and a tuning fork. I felt armed and ready for my next assignment: Internship and Residency.

After medical school graduation, you officially have an M.D. after your name and can be called "doctor." There is also a classic joke about medical school: "What do you call the student doctor at the bottom of the class?" The answer? "Doctor." Most patients will never know what your rank was in your medical school, and the subject rarely ever comes up post-graduation.

Simply surviving and making it through medical school is pretty much all anyone cares about. But there's an adage in medicine, "Don't get sick in July." That is because July is the month when medical students become intern doctors, with maximum responsibility for patient care at a time when their knowledge is at its lowest. A lot of mistakes can occur in July.

It is a pretty heady experience the first time you are addressed by the staff or a patient as a physician, no longer a student doctor, and initially, it makes you work harder. But, over time, the same fatigue that plagued you in medical school begins to exhibit as an intern and resident. The hours are long, the work is often thankless, and you can tire from the seeming lack of ability to heal or actually help your patients.

Some patients want to get better, some don't, preferring to complain about their illness and seek medical care incessantly. Some patients' entire identity is wrapped up in some diagnosis they have received at some point in their lives. Other patients exhibit signs of "Munchausen's Syndrome," which is when patients *create* their illness to receive attention and care from the medical establishment. Other patients have a revolving door to the hospital or clinic, and some never leave the hospital, ending their stay in the morgue.

Over time, the work can be overwhelming, unfulfilling, and physically and mentally exhausting. Occasionally, you bond with patients in a way that makes it all worthwhile. Training to be a full-fledged physician, depending on the specialty you choose, can be based in the hospital, an outpatient clinic, or, most commonly, both. Your choice of specialty may determine where in the U.S. you complete your training.

Because my husband was employed in a career and job he wanted to keep, I applied to internship and residency programs only in my hometown, where I had attended medical school. This is an unusual thing to do. Most physicians, looking for their advanced specialty training after medical school, apply throughout the country to match somewhere - anywhere, really. I was not in a position to move due to my family circumstances, so I only applied for training in my backyard. I was matched to an excellent internship and residency program in one of my area's top community hospitals.

The residency I attended was headed up by the Chief of Medicine, a delightful and jovial older British man who was an incredible human and leader of newly minted doctors. Dr. Britain did his level best to make some moments more enjoyable during residency. He went above and beyond to make us feel like family and hosted barbecues at his beautiful home. He was known for his beaming smile, frequent compliments on our work, and gentle guidance when course correction was needed. He made our experience in residency so much better and more rewarding.

Internship and Residency, after completing four years of medical school, or five in my case, can be brutal. Training can last for nearly an additional decade, depending on the specialty you have chosen. At the time I trained, there was no restriction on work hours for residents, so 100-hour work weeks were routine and expected. The fatigue and overwhelm that accompany medical training, including the constant need to learn new and vital information, are hard to describe.

At the same time, you are learning so much new information, you are not able to sleep much, and meals can be infrequent. Another adage in medical training is, "Eat when you can, sleep when you can." You are also often required to perform dangerous procedures when you're so tired you don't know if you can continue. It makes for an interesting dynamic, and not always a good one. But I can say that some of the best learning I have had has been in the last hours of the week, when I was so exhausted and not sure I could carry on for another minute. Somehow, your adrenaline kicks in and you get the job done.

These stories from my residency training program are just a few of the amazing interactions I had with my patients.

Chapter 17
Dr. Death

In residency, I was quickly given a nickname of "Doctor Death." I was given that name because I was unafraid of both talking with my patients about death and being with them as they transitioned to the afterworld. To me, it seemed like both a high honor - and a matter of respect - to stay with my patients as they died. I think initially the nickname by my peers was a slight. But over time, my colleagues began to ask me to counsel them about how to talk about death and dying with their patients. I was even asked by Dr. Britain to give a formal presentation to my colleagues on the topic.

I have no idea where this comfort with death and dying came from in me. I certainly wasn't religious or able to ascribe this activity to some spiritual ideology. I simply found it highly rewarding to be with my patients during their hour of need and time of transition.

One such patient was David. He presented to the ER for severe headaches, so bad that he was no longer able to perform his high-tech job. Before presenting to the hospital, he had seen both his primary care physician and a neurologist for his headaches. Both physicians had essentially "blown him off," giving him scripts for pain pills, but no imaging. They said his headaches were due to the stress of his job and encouraged him to take time off work.

David was in his early 40s, married with a beautiful wife, and two adorable children. When I met David, he was sitting propped up in his hospital bed with sunglasses on to shield his sensitive eyes from the light. He was surrounded by his family. I approached the bed and introduced myself to David and his family. I sat with them for over an hour and began to formulate my "differential diagnosis," or a list of potential explanations for his headaches.

I took a detailed history from David, and his wife gave helpful additional information when David couldn't remember everything accurately. In addition to memory problems, David's speech was occasionally slurred, making it difficult to interpret what he was trying to say.

The more they spoke, the more worried I became. I began to make a comprehensive list of all the tests and studies I would need to order for him to work up his worsening headaches. I took a detailed history and performed a physical examination on David, looking for signs that might point me to the etiology of his headaches. When I finished, I said, "David, I am going to go now and discuss your headaches with my boss, Dr. Neurology. I will be back soon to let you know our plan."

"Thank you, Dr. Casper, we really appreciate your time," David's wife offered. As I prepared to leave, David gave me the thumbs-up sign and a slightly crooked smile.

I left David's room and searched for my attending physician to present this case to him. Dr. Neurology was a brilliant and kind man, very respectful of doctors in training, and always willing to listen and provide guidance. I found him in the Doctor's Dining Room (DDR) having lunch. I pulled up a chair and sat next to him. "Get some lunch, Liz, and we can talk about the case," he offered. As a resident, I was not supposed to eat there, but Dr. Neurology's permission was all I needed to grab a salad and a coffee.

Before I dove into my lunch, I presented David's case to Dr. Neurology, emphasizing the lack of workup he had received as an outpatient. "What do you want to do, Liz?" he asked after I completed my presentation and between bites of his lunch.

"Honestly, he probably only needs one study, an MRI with contrast of his brain," I offered, assuming Dr. Neurology was thinking the same thing I was.

"I agree, great job, Liz," he replied as he continued to eat his lunch. I felt embarrassed at his kind words for a simple solution that most anyone would have thought of. Anyone, apparently, except the two community physicians David had seen before admission.

I quickly finished my meal and excused myself from the table. I went back to the wards and ordered the brain MRI for David. Afterwards, I went back into his room to let them know the plan and obtain consent. "What are we looking for, Dr. Casper?" David asked me point-blank.

This is when it can feel very uncomfortable for a doctor in training, and often, patients will only want to speak to the attending physician. David and his family were different. They seemed to trust me implicitly and were content receiving pertinent medical information from me alone.

"David, we are looking for an explanation for your headaches," I responded. "We need to rule out things like cancer, a benign tumor, multiple sclerosis, etc. An MRI will give us a lot of information," I finished as I handed them a stack of papers and consents for David to sign. They were so grateful for any test to help solve the mystery of David's headaches. His wife hugged me as I left the room.

At that time in medicine, imaging studies were read by radiologists who were physically in the hospital, and it usually took 24 hours or more for a result. Before I left for the day, I placed an order for the MRI and asked to have the imaging study read as soon as possible. I hoped the results would be available the next day to discuss with David.

The next morning, I came to work early to check on David's MRI. I logged onto the computer at the nurse's station and braced myself for the results. Unfortunately, my hunch had been right, and David had a mass in his head the size of a baseball, presumed cancer. The tumor was most likely a Glioblastoma Multiforme (GBM), the most deadly kind. I peeked into David's room and was happy to see his family had gone home, and he was sleeping peacefully in his room.

I found Dr. Neurology and discussed the MRI results with him. He, too, was not surprised, but disheartened (as I was) at the months-long lack of outpatient care David had received before admission. "Liz, I think you are up for the task of telling David about the MRI results," he stated. "The family raved about you when I met them yesterday. Please find out if they would like to proceed with a biopsy."

Later that morning, I met up with David and his wife. I sat on a chair next to his bed and made sure that I wasn't "talking over them" as I gave them the devastating news. "David, we have the results of your MRI," I stated. "The news is not good, and it looks like you most likely have brain cancer. There is a small chance that this lesion - the size of a baseball - is benign, but not likely."

"What do we do now?" David's beautiful wife asked me as David gave me a blank stare. I couldn't tell if he understood what I had just relayed to them.

"Well, our next step would be to do a biopsy, but that is an invasive procedure with risks. But to get a definitive diagnosis, we need to get tissue from the mass," I replied. I turned back to David to search for direction from him.

"Let's do the biopsy," he said as tears streamed down his wife's face.

David did have the biopsy, and the mass was indeed GBM, the most common, aggressive, and deadly kind of brain cancer you can get. All I could think about was how unlucky David was. His cancer was growing exceptionally quickly, and his neurological status began to deteriorate as the days passed in the hospital. David decided against further brain surgery, which really wasn't a good option given the size and location of his tumor.

David further declined radiation and chemotherapy, the only other two options available at that time, both with dismal outcomes for this type of cancer. David chose quality of life over quantity of time remaining.

The decision was made by Dr. Neurology and me to not discharge David, but rather provide supportive, palliative care in the hospital. We knew he didn't have long to live and called Hospice to assist with his hospital care and family support. One morning, on my usual visit to see all of my patients before rounds, I popped my head into David's room. He was resting alone, so I pulled up a chair and sat close to his bed. "David, can you hear me?" I asked in a whispered tone.

David opened his eyes slowly and said, "Yes, I hear you. I don't think I have long now." We both knew he was right. As he shut his eyes, I wiped tears from my face. David and his beautiful young family reminded me of my own and illuminated how fragile we, and this life, are. I reached for his hand and squeezed it gently before I left the room.

David died two days later, with his wife and me at his side. Once again, Dr. Death was with her patient as he transitioned, a responsibility I never took lightly. His wife asked me to come to the funeral, which I did. David was a pillar of his community, and the funeral was packed. His light was snuffed out far too soon.

Chapter 18
A Medical Mystery

My internship and residency were a blend of outpatient and inpatient work. For being a community program, it was considered quite academic and rigorous. Dr. Britain, our chief of medicine, was world-renowned in his specialty and expected his physicians-in-training to take the rigors of academia seriously.

As is common in hospital work, there can be some really challenging cases and vexing diagnoses. Oftentimes, there is a bit of competitiveness to see who on the service will figure out the medical mystery first, regardless of whose patient it was. I was about to get one of those new admissions on my service, and I would be the primary physician on the case. My training program rarely had medical students rotate through, so most of the work - both intellectual and physical - would be all mine. An exciting and terrifying possibility.

This particular rotation - in the Intensive Care Unit (ICU) - was reported to be one of the most difficult in our training. I approached the ICU on my first day with trepidation, mild excitement, and terror. The ICU was filled with dings, beeps, cardiac monitors, ventilators, feeding tubes, IVs, and more. Most of the patients were critically ill and knocking on death's door. The new patient assigned to me was no different.

The ICU was run by two critical care specialists: an intense but irreverent middle-aged white guy, and a younger, serious-as-a-heart-attack black man. He rarely cracked a smile in the four weeks we worked together, but he was considered one of the smartest doctors on staff. Most of us residents took his off-putting personality in stride, as we adored the learning he would occasionally impart on us. He did not suffer fools, or really much of anything. He hailed from Stanford, and getting facetime with him, regardless of his countenance or mood, was a sought-after activity for the learning it would impart.

A new patient had come into our ICU for further workup from an outlying hospital. He had been hospitalized there without improvement for over a month. The prior hospital had done as much of a thorough workup on him as they could, but a diagnosis had eluded them. The patient was getting worse by the day, and upon transfer to our hospital, he was admitted directly to the ICU.

The patient was a 29-year-old Indian man from Bombay. He was a software coder and had been brought into the U.S. recently on a "fast track VISA" to work for one of our local high-tech pariahs. This meant that he did not have the proper medical screening and quarantine for potential third-world illnesses, as is required for admission to the U.S. He had "slipped through the cracks" of our immigration system, *intentionally.*

In 1990, the U.S. government began a program called the H-1B visa program with the passage of the Immigration Act of 1990. The patient, named Navi, had only been in the US for less than one month before he became too sick to go to work. He lived in a two-bedroom apartment with five other guys from India, also coders at the same high-tech company. None of them had been screened for any illnesses before they had come to work in the U.S., as their skills were needed "imminently," according to his employer.

By the time Navi was transferred to our hospital, he was rapidly intubated and placed on a ventilator, making my interview plans obsolete. I was now relegated to sleuthing through the inches-thick paper medical chart from the outlying hospital, talking to his roommates when I could, and talking with the HR department of his employer. My job was to do my homework and begin to assemble the pieces of the puzzle to present to Dr. Stanford.

Although not nearly as sexy, being a doctor can be pretty much like being a detective. Sometimes, the facts and the physician's clinical acumen lead to a win, and saving of the patient, sometimes not. Often, you are racing against time before the unknown illness kills your patient.

Of course, if you have some medical training and are reading this, you are certainly thinking of tuberculosis as I was. The problem was that all of the usual tests for TB had been performed at the prior hospital, and all had been negative. But if it walks like a duck, quacks like a duck, you get the picture. I was relatively certain that TB was the only realistic potential diagnosis. But it appeared that all of the investigations in his month-long hospitalization before our ICU admission had come up negative. It was time for some creative medical thinking to solve Navi's case.

Tuberculosis is an infectious disease caused by the bug Mycobacterium tuberculosis, and is primarily seen in low- and middle-income countries, such as India. It is generally rare to find it in the U.S. population. TB is spread from person to person by airborne droplets through coughing, speaking, or sneezing. Symptoms include a bloody cough, fever, night sweats, and weight loss. It appeared from Navi's medical record from the prior hospital that he had initially presented with these symptoms. TB can also be deadly, killing over 1.5 million people worldwide each year.

The care team in the ICU rounded on Navi every morning, and we watched in frustration as his condition worsened by the day. One morning, while rounding with Dr. Stanford and the entire team, he mentioned that he recalled an obscure test (couldn't remember the name) performed on the cerebrospinal fluid (CSF) to diagnose difficult-to-find TB. This was a test we had yet to perform.

He recalled that the only hospital lab that performed the test for him, ages ago, and while he was still in his training at Stanford, was Denver Jewish, located in Denver, Colorado. He suggested that I call them to further investigate the current availability of the test, so I did.

I spoke to the head of the lab at Denver Jewish who told me that the test was called the "adenosine deaminase test," and was performed on the CSF. He let me know that they hadn't performed the test in years, but still could. He said it was a rarely-used test that could definitively diagnose TB when all other diagnostic tests had failed to reveal the pathogen. He remembered Dr. Stanford from working with him years earlier and asked me to give my regards to him.

I reported my findings from Denver Jewish to Dr. Stanford, and he gave me the highest compliment ever for a doctor in training: I would get to perform the lumbar puncture on our intubated patient in the ICU, a challenging procedure in the best of circumstances. I simultaneously felt honored and terrified.

A lumbar puncture, also known as a spinal tap, is a medical procedure where a long, hollow needle is inserted into the lower spine (the lumbar region) to collect CSF for evaluation. Typically, the patient lies on their side in a fetal position to make the intervertebral space more available. Or, they sit up in bed, hunched over. An intubated Navi was unable to do either, making it very difficult to do the work. It took several nurses, Dr. Stanford, and me to complete the procedure. Somehow, we successfully finished the job and sent off Navi's CSF to Denver Jewish for testing.

The test took a week to come back, but the results were well worth the wait. Navi did indeed have systemic, devastating, multidrug-resistant TB, located in odd areas of his body outside of the pulmonary norms. By this point, and having been hospitalized for nearly two months, one in the ICU, Navi was going to be difficult to treat.

The cultures finally came back as well, and we tailored a quadruple drug regimen to treat the result of his cultures. After a couple of weeks on the meds, he was able to be extubated and moved to a medical floor. He stayed in the hospital for an additional six months until he died.

This whole situation was tragedy piled upon tragedy, brought on by crushing corporate greed and the breaking of the H-1B U.S. immigration rules. Three of Navi's roommates also contracted TB from him and ended up in the hospital. But fortunately, they were able to benefit - and live - due to the knowledge we acquired from Navi. The whole situation was complicated by the fact that these men did not have any health insurance, either, leaving the hospital to foot the bill.

Navi's bill alone for the hospital was well over two million dollars at the time he died.

Chapter 19
Detective in the ICU

The ICU was one of the most intimidating and interesting places in the hospital, except for the OR. A lot went down there, and things change at a moment's notice, so there is rarely a dull moment. On one of my overnight shifts, I was unable to sleep, so I decided to roam around the ICU. A crusty older ICU nurse introduced herself to me and said, "Dr. Casper, if you want to do well here, you will do whatever we, the nurses, tell you to do. We are the ones who *really* run this place."

Good to know, I thought to myself. I found the ICU nurse's approach a little off-putting, but after I completed another four weeks in the ICU, I can honestly say that I succeeded *because* of the nurses, not despite them. They were a wealth of knowledge, and imminently more available than the physician attendings.

I watched in mild amusement as my male colleagues did not heed the nurse's advice, and they paid dearly for it. Nurses hate any arrogance from a physician in training, and they can quickly put you in your place. They are often a constant reminder of how little you know at the beginning of residency.

As a physician in residency training, nurses can absolutely make your life miserable, and getting on their good side early is a really good idea. "Good side" means that you do your job well, listen to them, follow their direction, and don't be cocky. If a nurse likes you, she or he might not wake you up in the middle of the night for an inconsequential patient question. If they don't like you or think you are egotistic, you suffer the consequences, get called more frequently, and get less sleep.

Earlier that day, I had been assigned to a new admission. He was a 24-year-old man in a coma, found unresponsive in his home by his girlfriend. He was intubated in the ER. I had spoken with the girlfriend, and she had no idea what had happened to John. She reported, to her knowledge, John did not drink alcohol or use recreational drugs. All of the studies and blood work that we had already performed had come back negative, including a comprehensive drug panel.

Another freaking medical mystery, I thought to myself as I took a seat outside his room and stared at the monitors in front of me. I was so tired, and I wasn't feeling very inspired or intelligent at that point. It was 3 a.m., so I decided to go back to bed and try to get a little sleep before my day began with the ICU team at 6 a.m. sharp. I walked back through the sterile hallways to the tiny residents' room where there are two single beds for my teammate and me to sleep.

To get back to the residents' quarters, I had to pass by the pediatric wing. I noticed the large painted jungle animals on the wall and remembered that John's girlfriend said he worked in a veterinary office. It suddenly occurred to me that he might have been exposed to some toxin while at work. I decided to pursue that rabbit hole the next morning. I reached the residents' room and flopped down on the tiny bed with a rubber pillow.

I quickly fell asleep, but was awakened soon thereafter by a helpful ICU nurse. She needed my permission to order a non-urgent medicine for a patient, which could have easily waited until later in the morning. Clearly, I still had some work to do with making inroads with the nurses to avoid these ridiculous interruptions to my brief attempt to get some shuteye. I approved her request for Tylenol for a patient I wasn't following, and did my best to get another hour of sleep before the day began.

The next morning, I prepared for rounds by doing some internet research on veterinary clinics. I learned that they use multiple "human" drugs on animals. I also learned that

Ketamine was often used as a sedative for veterinary surgery, but it can be diverted and used as a recreational drug for those who are willing to take the risk.

At that time, Ketamine was used for both humans and animals as part of anesthesia and for pain relief. Ketamine also delivers a dissociative state and imparts a "high" to those who use it. Ketamine later received FDA approval for outpatient use in humans, but at that time, it was strictly regulated and only available in hospitals, surgery centers, operating rooms, and veterinary clinics.

Ketamine at low doses provides euphoria, altered perception, and mild disassociation. At higher doses, users can feel completely detached from reality. When taken at very high or toxic doses, Ketamine can cause delirium and seizures. Severe overdosing can result in respiratory depression requiring intubation, hypotension, and bradycardia, as seen in our patient. Acute overuse of ketamine, as I suspected with John, can cause swelling of the brain and coma. Additionally, it can cause kidney failure, liver failure, and destruction of the skeletal muscles.

I felt pressure to solve John's mystery and to help him get better. Later that morning, I presented my Ketamine idea at rounds in the ICU. "Dr. Stanford, I have a hypothesis about what may be causing John's coma," I said with as much confidence as I could muster in front of the large group standing outside John's ICU room.

"Oh, really, Dr. Casper, do tell," Dr. Stanford said to everyone as he looked around at the group. He continued, "Our sleuth here thinks she has solved our daily mystery in the ICU!"

All eyes were on me at that point, so I blurted out, "Sir, I think he has overdosed on Ketamine."

"Ketamine? Really? Please do explain your reasoning," he replied.

"Well, he works for a vet clinic that uses Ketamine. I called the clinic earlier this morning, and the veterinarian there said that they were missing a large amount of Ketamine." I continued, "Our standard drug testing panel does not include Ketamine, so I think we should test him for it."

At that moment, I managed to get a look of surprise and delight from Dr. Stanford, a rarity. Clearly, he appreciated my sleuthing and said so in front of the group. This only motivated me to work harder to find the answer.

After rounds, I ordered John's blood test, and the result came back positive for a toxic dose of Ketamine. As you might imagine, a dose of Ketamine for a horse would be very different from a dose for a human. My patient, new to the veterinary world, had diverted the medication and mistakenly taken a massive dose, leaving him in a coma.

After another week in the ICU and a couple doses of flumazenil, John woke up and was eventually able to be weaned off the ventilator. Unfortunately, due to the total dose of Ketamine that John took and the prolonged time spent in a coma, he did not ever fully recover and definitely lost more than a few IQ points.

At the end of my ICU rotation, Dr. Stanford told me that I was one of the best doctors-in-training detectives that he had ever worked with. High, high praise from the man made of stone.

Chapter 20
Ice Cream Charlie

Early in my medical training as a resident and child rearing, my husband and I lived in a poor, urban environment. It was literally all we could afford, so we tried to make the best of a sketchy situation. We endeavored to assimilate with our neighbors and make friends. One such activity that promoted a group gathering "in the hood" was a visit from Charlie.

Charlie was a regular in our neighborhood, driving an old ice cream truck daily past our home. If we were home, our children would hear the jingly, carnival music emanating from his refrigerated truck, and would beg us for a treat from Charlie. His truck was adorned in a rainbow of colors and big pictures displaying the treats inside. "Pop Goes the Weasel" and "The Entertainer" were heard from blocks away.

Our kids always alerted my husband and me to the oncoming treat truck, causing daily excitement and shouts for ice cream all summer long. Generally, we complied, and Charlie would often park in front of our house as he spread good cheer to all of the neighborhood children.

Ice cream Charlie wasn't young, yet he also wasn't old. It was hard to tell his age, but he looked like he had had a tough life. Regardless, he greeted every kid - and parent - with a big smile and wave, even remembering names. He handed out samples of ice cream to the kids and served summer happiness with each visit. Charlie was a fixture in our neighborhood and our children's young lives. He was an "urban ice cream legend," and to our young kids, he was a hero.

One day, during my general surgery rotation with Dr. Smith, my attending indicated that we needed to "run an errand" before starting our next case in the OR. Always wanting to seem professional and detached, I did not ask him where we were going or why. I dutifully followed him off the surgical ward to the elevators and downstairs after he pushed the elevator button for "Basement," an area of the hospital I had rarely been to before. I did not know our reason for going there.

During our elevator descent, my boss turned to me and said, "We have to stop by the morgue." I knew the hospital had a morgue, but I had never been there before. I wasn't sure why he was being asked to go there, but I kept any further questions to myself, so as not to seem squeamish or too curious and unprofessional.

We reached the basement and walked down a long hallway, brightly lit and sterile-looking. At the end of the hall was the morgue, and the minute he opened the door, the smell of formaldehyde assaulted my nose. I held back the reflex to cough or plug my nose and took quick, short breaths as we entered the room.

We walked through the morgue and located the hospital mortician. "Hello, Dr. Smith, thank you for coming. We have a new body we need to pronounce," said the mortician. Dr. Smith and the man shook hands and started to walk together. I was not introduced, and I felt my presence there was unnecessary. We walked through several rooms to locate the newly deceased person, covered with a white sheet, concealing their identity.

We walked toward the table together. "You know, this guy was supposed to be an added emergency surgery on my schedule this morning for an exploratory laparotomy," Dr. Smith stated to the mortician, identifying the patient as a man for the first time. "I decided to come down here myself to see what happened to him."

"Well, sir, let's just say that he's had a *very* bad morning," the mortician replied.

"Yes, I can see that," Dr. Smith stated in a sarcastic tone, as he looked around the morgue filled with dead people covered with white sheets. "This ain't no OR!" he replied with a grim smile.

"Rather than making it to your OR, he is here with me," the mortician replied. "The ER thought his broken bones were the extent of his problems, but I've uncovered the internal bleeding of his spleen that caused his death," he finished.

Once the three of us surrounded the body, the mortician pulled back the sheet to reveal the patient's head. As he did so, I let out a loud gasp. On the table was Ice Cream Charlie, whom my kids had just purchased ice cream from the day before. I couldn't believe who I was looking at. I began to feel nauseated, and I felt my heart begin to beat faster.

Surely, there must be some mix-up? Did Charlie have a twin brother? I thought to myself as the reality of what I was witnessing started to settle in. I was horrified and speechless at that moment.

"Dr. Casper, is everything okay?" Dr. Smith asked me, seemingly genuinely concerned as he gazed at my face, which was unable to conceal my shock.

"Well, sir, I know this man," I blurted out, then immediately regretted divulging anything personal about myself at that moment.

"I'm sorry to hear that," Dr. Smith replied. He looked confused as to how I would know this now-dead, scruffy man, covered in blood, lying on the table.

My knees felt weak as I turned my attention to the mortician. "Sir, do you know *how* this man died?" I asked as my lips began to tremble.

"Yes, he drives an ice cream truck. He was T-boned by a high-speed driver in the middle of an intersection on his route," the mortician answered.

"Do you know *what* intersection?" I asked, as I started to feel sick.

"Yes, I believe that it was at the intersection of 10th Avenue and Washington Street this morning," the mortician replied.

I was stunned. That was "our" intersection - in a bad part of town. *You have to be kidding me. What are the chances? I thought to myself.*

At this point, Dr. Smith performed the required steps to officially pronounce Charlie deceased, listing the cause of death as internal bleeding from trauma. He finished his job by replacing the white sheet over his head.

Internal bleeding is a major cause of death in car accidents, often resulting from blunt trauma or penetrating injuries during a crash. It occurs when the blood vessels rupture inside the body, leading to blood loss that's often not immediately visible, but can quickly become a major problem. Common bleeding sites are the spleen (as in Charlie's case), liver, aortic tears, or pelvic injuries.

Symptoms like shock, low blood pressure, or organ failure can rapidly develop. In a car (or in an ice cream truck) accident, internal bleeding is frequently caused by high-impact collisions, crushing injuries, or seatbelt trauma. If there is a delay in the diagnosis of internal bleeding following a traumatic car accident, death can rapidly occur. Head injuries remain the leading cause of death from car accidents, but internal bleeding is a significant contributor to death, especially in high-speed, or T-bone impacts, as in Charlie's case.

Dr. Smith and I left the morgue and started our day of general surgery: hernia repairs, gall bladder removal, colon cancer removal, etc. He did not ask me any questions about Charlie, and I did not offer any information about my performance in the morgue. For Dr. Smith, pronouncing the ice cream hero dead was nothing more than "doing his job" and "all in a day's work." To me, it hit differently, and I spent most of my day thinking about how I was going to tell my children. Later, in between cases in the OR, I called my husband with the news, and we decided to tell the kids together at the "right time," at some point in the future.

The day Charlie died, I got home from my day in surgery very late and after the kids were in bed. The next day that I had off from work, we took the kids out for ice cream at Baskin-Robbins. They asked why we couldn't get our ice cream from Charlie. This started the difficult conversation about life and death, and no more ice cream trucks in front of our house.

While finishing our ice cream, my oldest child summed up the situation perfectly: Charlie was now in heaven, where he could eat ice cream every day without having to drive a truck. My younger child found a great deal of comfort with that explanation from their older sibling, easing the emotional roller coaster my husband and I worried they would be on.

There is a lot of wisdom in very young people. And in the end, I think I took the news of Charlie's death the hardest out of all of us.

Chapter 21

Mr. Addict

In my tenure as an intern, I was assigned again to the Intensive Care Unit for a third, month-long rotation. The rotation in the ICU was considered one of the most taxing, and few of us wanted to be there more than once in our first year of residency training. Somehow, I lucked out with three months of ICU work in my first year of residency.

The patients in the ICU were very complex; the technology was overwhelming; and the teaching could be sparse. A very high-pressure environment at just the time that our knowledge base as interns was the most shallow. To put it bluntly, it was hard work and long hours, often leaving you feeling impotent and inept. Most of us just hoped to survive, and not cause harm or kill a patient.

The activity and complexity of the patients in the ICU are often exacerbated by other issues, such as ethical issues. The most difficult cases occur when the family is absent and the patient is unable to communicate for themselves, usually because they were intubated. Mr. Addict, an IV heroin drug user, was one such case.

IV drug use is risky from several perspectives, with sepsis, abscesses, heart infections, HIV, and Hepatitis B & C commonplace. Additionally, overdosing is a very real risk, with 70% of all drug overdose deaths as a result of IV opioid use. The current statistics regarding IV drug use in the USA, at the time of authoring this book, are staggering and shocking. Approximately four million people (1.5%) are addicted to heroin, fentanyl, and methamphetamine, the most commonly used drugs, followed by cocaine and ketamine.

The most common outcome of heroin use, as in our patient, is addiction. It develops rapidly with heroin use due to its highly habit-forming nature. Short-term effects include euphoria, sedation, and pain relief. With repeated use, tolerance builds, requiring higher doses of heroin to achieve the same effect, which significantly increases the risk of overdose.

Many addicts report diminishing effects of the drug with repeated use, and many are always on the quest to re-achieve the profound euphoria they felt with their *first use* of the drug. Continued use of opioids delivers diminishing returns to the user due to tolerance. Recovery is possible with treatment using a drug like methadone, but relapse rates exceed 50%.

The drug epidemic affects 60 million Americans overall, and young males most commonly. Unfortunately, the epidemic continues to rise each year. IV drug use is extremely risky, under the best of circumstances, with infection being one of the most common adverse outcomes due to reusing or sharing needles.

Approximately 20% of all HIV cases are caused by IV drug use. IV drug use can also introduce pathogens like bacteria and fungi into the bloodstream, making delicate tissues, like a heart valve, at great risk of infection and "blowing out." Oftentimes, antibiotics are of little use for a heart valve infection, and surgical valve replacement may be required to save the addict's life.

Other sequelae from IV drug use are overdoses, killing hundreds of thousands of Americans every year. Additionally, one of the worst complications, save death, is necrotizing fasciitis, a condition resulting from injecting drugs via "skin popping" in an enclosed space like a muscle bundle. What is probably the most discouraging statistic is that less than 10% of drug abusers ever receive treatment for their disease.

Mr. Addict had been in our ICU several times before, always for the same thing: sepsis and infection of a heart valve. This condition, known as infective endocarditis, was a result of his continued IV drug use and from reusing or sharing needles. Mr. Addict's drug of choice was heroin, but in past hospitalizations, he admitted to using "anything he could get his hands on," when necessary to feed his addiction.

Mr. Addict was 26 years old, unemployed for his life, without a home, and without health insurance. He had had three prior mitral heart valve replacement surgeries at our institution alone. This is a massive surgery with severe morbidity and prolonged hospital stays. And when he was well enough to leave the ICU, he would stay on the hospital wards for an additional month or two before being discharged back to the streets. Once there, he would restart his IV drug use, only to be readmitted soon thereafter with the same diagnosis again and again.

Surgical heart valve replacement is a modern-era miracle, allowing patients to live generally healthy lives after surgery. The valve replacement is meant to be a one-time procedure, not a repeatable intervention. Heart valves - at that time in medicine - could either be made from pigs (biological tissue) or metal (a mechanical, artificial valve). Both valves have their advantages and disadvantages. The choice of which one to implant is made by the cardiovascular surgeon based upon the circumstances of the patient receiving the valve.

Mr. Addict had only received tissue valves because you have to take blood thinners to receive the more durable mechanical valve. This was something Mr. Addict would not, or could not do, as a homeless man. So, he repeatedly received tissue valves, which don't require blood thinning, but are very vulnerable to infection. IV drug use is the perfect entrée for repeat infection of one's heart valves.

Each valve replacement surgery on Mr. Addict had required open heart surgery, a massively invasive surgery with known morbidity and mortality. After each surgery, he would spend time in the ICU and the wards, often totaling 90 days or more with each admission. Mr. Addict was lucky to be alive.

Late one day, as I was preparing to leave the hospital, I was asked to take Mr. Addict for his admission to the ICU. This meant hours of work and missing dinner with my family and my children's bedtime. I was exhausted, but that didn't matter. When Dr. Stanford assigns you a patient, the only acceptable response is to do the work without complaint or accommodation.

When I met Mr. Addict, he was fresh out of surgery to replace his latest mitral valve, unconscious, and on a ventilator. The majority of the work I had to do revolved around reading two feet of prior admission chart notes and transferring the last admission's orders to this admission.

Mr. Addict had a revolving door in our hospital, and over the previous two years, it appeared that no one had ever had a conversation with him about his lifestyle or future. His hospital bills, by the time I met him, had exceeded five million dollars in total. Here he was, again, getting top-tier care and a massive medical procedure, with no personal responsibility or accountability. And, no ability to pay.

The more I read in his chart, the more frustrated I became, thinking about how many people could have been helped by five million dollars of free hospital medical care. Why, why, *why* was everyone involved in Mr. Addict's care only concerned about *what* antibiotic to prescribe, *what* heart valve to replace, or *what* skilled facility wouldn't accept him this time upon discharge? I was shocked and appalled at the waste of resources and lack of attention to the ethical issues that were raised in his case.

I performed a brief physical exam on Mr. Addict, who was unconscious and on a ventilator, making notes of the copious lesions on his limbs, the remnant of skin popping his drug of choice. Addicts begin to skin pop after they have "used up" all of their available veins, and it is a harbinger of a hardened addict. His skin was pale and gray, his limbs emaciated from the lack of nutrition, and his face was weathered from being housed on the streets. He appeared much older than his stated age.

After I had completed my work for the night with Mr. Addict, I looked around the ICU for Dr. Stanford. I hoped he would back me up and endorse the plan I had in mind. I found Dr. Stanford sitting in front of the monitors outside another patient's ICU room, deep in thought. I sat down next to him and waited for him to acknowledge me. After a few minutes, he turned to me and said, "So, Dr. Casper, is our drug addict settled in?"

"Hi, Dr. Stanford, yes, I've finished with Mr. Addict. He is tucked in for the night," I replied. We discussed the case, and to no surprise, he knew the patient well. Dr. Stanford had supervised his care during several prior ICU admissions. "Dr. Stanford, what do you think about getting an ethics committee review of his case?" I asked confidently. I was surprised, however, that he had not suggested this idea for an ethics consult himself on Mr. Addict's prior admissions, given how practical he was.

"Why would you do that, Dr. Casper?" he asked with a quizzical look. "He just got out of surgery and is still intubated. What's the rush?"

"Well, it seems appropriate given that he seems to have a second home here in this hospital. He keeps getting admitted for the same thing; keeps getting a new heart valve each time; and apparently refuses to get help and stop his IV drug use," I replied.

"Agreed, but he's only 26, Liz," he stated.

"Yes, he is. But sir, with all due respect, this hospital has provided five million dollars of medical care to him with no improvement in his outcome. He's just received his fourth heart valve at our institution alone. That money could help a lot of other uninsured people who are motivated to get well," I replied.

"Interesting perspective. I'm not sure I agree with you, but okay, go ahead and order the ethics consult," he finished. He turned his attention back to the monitors, clearly indicating our conversation was over. Before I left the hospital for the night, I placed an order in Mr. Addict's chart for a formal ethics committee consultation.

I met with the ethics team the next day and explained the situation. They had prepared for our meeting by reviewing Mr. Addict's extensive chart beforehand. The first question I was asked by the head of the committee - a Chaplain - was *why* they weren't consulted earlier at prior admissions. I, of course, had to let them know that this was the first time that I was meeting Mr. Addict, but I indeed felt he needed to be seen by them. *Better late than never*, I thought to myself.

In the end, the ethics committee decided it was time to stop providing this inequitable, free care to Mr. Addict. As one final stopgap measure, when he was extubated, awake, and coherent, we met with him as a team with Dr. Stanford and the ethics committee. He was offered the opportunity to go to free, inpatient, rehab treatment to get clean and sober, once and for all. He declined, *again*.

Mr. Addict was finally able to be discharged after another two months in our hospital, but to the best of my knowledge, he was never readmitted to our institution.

Chapter 22
The Psychiatric Ward

When you graduate from medical school and have completed your first post-graduate year of internship, you can apply for a limited license in certain states. This allows you to work as an independent physician outside the confines of your residency program, if time and the program allow.

Some programs do not allow you to pick up extra work. But if they do, this additional employment opportunity permits you to make a little extra money, as the compensation from residency training approximates minimum wage. Money is usually very tight while in your residency training as the pay is low, and student loans from medical school are now due for repayment.

Many of us in my residency program sought extra shifts and work to supplement our income. Post-graduate training for physicians significantly underpays for the job and hours expected of you. If you have any time left in your day or week, you might consider picking up extra shifts or assignments for additional pay. As I had two children by that point, in need of expensive childcare, my husband and I decided the tradeoff of time with my family for extra income was worth it. In 20/20 hindsight, I am not sure it was worth the sacrifice.

One of the opportunities I had in my second year of residency was to admit patients to the psychiatric ward of the hospital I worked in. This assignment was done after hours, and I was paid a nominal amount. I would admit these patients for the attending psychiatrist, who would see the patient the next day. My job was to "tuck in" the patient for the night so that the attending would not have to come to the hospital themselves in the evening. Each intake could take hours, and the pay was minimal ($75), but at least it was something.

The psychiatric ward of our hospital was located on the sixth floor. Once you exited the elevator, you were met with locked metal doors in all directions. This was in contrast to the "regular wards," where other patients reside in the building without locks and security. On my first evening of working in the psychiatric unit, I took the elevator to floor 6. Once there, I realized that my regular hospital ID would not grant me access to the locked doors, so I rang the call button.

"Psychiatric ward, how can I help you?" a voice asked through an intercom.

"Hi, this is Dr. Casper. I'm here to admit a patient named Andrew for Dr. Psychiatry," I replied.

A loud buzzer rang, and one of the heavy metal doors unlocked, granting me access to the ward.

Once on the unit, I walked down a long hallway toward what appeared to be the nurses' station. There were patients in hospital gowns walking up and down the corridor, many acting very erratically. Some made gestures at me as I passed, and some were talking to someone that no one else could see. I heard shouts and sobbing coming from the various rooms as I passed by. It felt 180 degrees different from the other hospital wards, and I wondered what awaited me.

I had never been to the psychiatric ward before, so I had little idea of what Andrew's admission would be like. After entering the ward and walking down the hall, I searched for the nurse's station. I finally found it, encased in locked glass, unlike the other nurses' stations in the hospital. As I approached the desk, I noticed a couple of fully armed policemen standing outside a patient's room adjacent to the nurses' station, #606. I approached the desk to ask about the whereabouts of my patient.

"Hi, I'm Dr. Casper," I repeated to the secretary. "I'm here to admit a patient named Andrew."

"Hi, Dr. Casper," she replied. "Come back here, there's a desk where you can work," she said as she pressed another buzzer and unlocked the door to grant me access to the nurses' station. I was impressed with the security and wondered why it was necessary in a hospital. It didn't take long for me to figure out the reason for such tight security.

I entered the door to the locked nurses' station and took my seat at the desk meant for me. I logged on to the computer and familiarized myself with Andrew's reason for admission. I learned that he was homeless, schizophrenic, a drug user, and HIV positive. He had been in our institution many times before and was now being admitted for worsening psychotic symptoms and violent outbursts. My job was to get him settled in for the night in preparation for meeting with Dr. Psychiatry the next day.

It took me about an hour to sift through Andrew's past hospitalizations and the current reason for admission. As it was after hours, and I had to miss dinner with my family to complete the work, I decided to get a snack from the ward's kitchen. Graham crackers, peanut butter, and cranberry juice were the familiar nutrition eaten by medical students, residents, and doctors alike. I spread the peanut butter on the cracker with a spoon, as knives - even plastic ones - were not allowed on the psych ward.

As I ate, I wondered what else was considered contraband on the unit. Later, I found out that just about everything was banned on the psych ward. Unstable psychiatric patients have an uncanny ability to turn most anything into something dangerous to themselves or others, like shoelaces, hairbrushes, and pens. Self-harm and harm to others were monitored 24/7 on the psych ward.

Once my belly was sated and Andrew's chart review complete, I began to look for his nurse. I found her at another nurse's desk and introduced myself. "Hi, I'm Dr. Casper, here to tuck in Andrew."

"Hi, Dr. Casper, Andrew is here for worsening psychotic symptoms. He is homeless and is unable to take his medicines regularly. He gets admitted when his symptoms cannot be controlled. He was making violent threats to others in the community, including some business owners, so he was brought here. He probably should be in jail again, but he is too sick to go there right now, as you will see. One of the policemen will join you for your time with him as he is quite unstable and potentially dangerous," she finished.

Oh, wow, a patient so violent that I need to have the police with me? I thought. *This is an interesting start to this new employment opportunity!*

I exited the glassed-in nurse's station and headed to the policemen guarding room #606. "Hi, sir, I am the physician who will be interviewing and examining Andrew," I said to the nearest cop. "I'm told that one of you will join me in the room?" I asked as I looked at both of them for clarification.

The closest cop turned to me and said, "Good luck with that, doc. I will join you, but don't expect much. He's in pretty bad shape."

The cop then pulled some keys out of his pocket and turned to unlock the door to Andrew's room. I hadn't realized that he was locked *in* the room and wondered why. It didn't take long to learn the answer.

"Andrew, there's a doctor here who needs to talk to you," the cop said loudly to Andrew as we entered his room. The room, in contrast to the other wards in the hospital, was completely different. It was empty, except for the bed without sheets or a pillow, and a bathroom without a door, a mirror, or a toilet seat. It looked like a prison cell housed within the hospital.

Andrew was curled up in a fetal position on the floor in the corner of the room, completely naked. He had totally disassembled the bare bed and had somehow managed to rip up the padding from his thin mattress, now scattered around the room. The cop and I approached Andrew slowly, so as to not aggravate the situation further.

"I'm not talking to anyone!" Andrew shouted back at the cop. He looked totally disheveled and malnourished. He had a haunting look to his face, with hollow eyes and sunken cheeks. His naked body was covered with dirt, and his hands and fingernails were black with filth from the streets. Andrew was 33 years old, but his life on the streets made him look almost elderly.

I stood at the door with the cop and wasn't sure what to do. Andrew had a history of violence and had been incarcerated innumerable times, both in jail and the psychiatric ward. I wasn't sure of my safety at that point, even with an armed police officer in the room.

"Andrew, where are your clothes?" the cop asked him before I could.

"I don't know, I lost them," Andrew replied, as we viewed his filthy clothes lying in a heap next to him on the floor. He seemed completely unaware of his surroundings.

"You need to get dressed so that the doctor can examine you," the cop stated loudly and firmly. "We will come back in a couple of minutes. Get dressed now, Andrew," he commanded in a stern voice as we left the room.

The cop and I exited Andrew's room and waited outside the door for a few minutes. I was trying to process *how* I was going to perform what I needed to do to admit Andrew. I was new to having a cop as a chaperone in my patient care. *How close should I get to Andrew? Do I dare try to touch him and complete a physical exam?* I wondered. I had to admit to myself that this was one hell of a way to make a little extra income.

A few minutes later, the cop and I entered Andrew's room again. This time, he was sitting completely naked on the bed with a pair of underwear on his head. "Andrew, where are your clothes now?" the cop asked.

"I don't have any clothes!" Andrew replied emphatically. At this point, I decided to intervene, in hopes of moving the situation along, as I was getting impatient with the circumstances I found myself in.

"Andrew, can you tell me *why* you are in the hospital?" I asked him from across the room.

"Because nobody believes me!" Andrew shouted back in an exasperated tone. "I'm being watched and controlled by the government! They want to kill me! You want to kill me, too!" He was agitated and erratic, and began to flail his emaciated arms around like a ballet dancer on crack.

"Andrew, I'm a doctor. I'm here to make sure you have everything you need tonight. Dr. Psychiatry will see you tomorrow morning," I replied.

"Don't touch me!" Andrew shouted at the cop and me from across the room. We were nowhere near him. At that point, Andrew began to have a full-on, unintelligible conversation with an invisible guest in the room.

I looked at the police officer and back at Andrew. I wasn't sure what to do at that point. Andrew had a propensity for violence, and he was instructing me to stay away from him. I decided to forego the physical exam and resort to the interview, safely from across the room.

"Andrew, do you know what year it is?" I asked.

After much thought, he replied, "1976." The year was actually 1999.

"And can you tell me who is President of the United States?" I continued.

"Nixon," Andrew answered without hesitation. Bill Clinton was the correct answer.

"Andrew, can I listen to your heart and lungs?" I asked, wondering if there was *anything* I could do to initiate a physical exam. I also wondered if I would even be paid for my care of Andrew if I couldn't perform a physical exam on him. At that time, a physical exam was a requirement for admission to the hospital and for the billing of my services. Nothing seemed to be a good idea at that point, and I felt like just going home and ending this encounter.

"No one is touching me!" he shouted back at me as he waved his arms around in the air, as if he was dismissing us from the room. "My body is a temple, and *no one* touches it." It was clear that Andrew was in the middle of an active psychotic episode, and my safety - even with the police by my side - could not be guaranteed.

At that point, I had realized that I probably wasn't going to perform a physical exam on Andrew, and his answers to my questions indicated that he was far from oriented to time and place. I acknowledged to myself that there was little I could do for him at that moment and decided to end our interview. I turned to the cop and said, "I think I'm done here, thank you for your time."

The cop and I left Andrew's room, and I headed back to the nurses' station to write my admission note and orders. I had a lot to learn about schizophrenia before I finished for the night and could go home to my family. As I wrote his note, I wondered if this extracurricular activity was actually worth it, when I acknowledged the paltry sum that I would receive in exchange for missing another evening with my family.

I studied up and learned a lot about Andrew's illness. Schizophrenia affects about 1% of the worldwide population, around 25 million people afflicted. It is usually diagnosed in young adults and is slightly more common in men. It is found more commonly in urban environments and is seen more often in minority groups. About 1.1 million new cases are diagnosed each year.

Schizophrenia is a complex mental health condition that varies widely among those afflicted. The illness is defined by hallucinations, hearing voices, delusions, and seeing or hearing things that others can't. The afflicted can also act paranoid or express ideas that seem disconnected from reality.

Schizophrenics are not inherently violent or dangerous. But their behavior is shaped by their environment and whether or not they are receiving appropriate medical care and medication. There are some good medications, but administering quality care to a homeless person at that time was challenging, to say the least. Unfortunately, many people with untreated schizophrenia cycle between hospital admissions and stints in jail or prison. Many schizophrenics are also addicted to drugs.

I finished up my admission note by ordering the appropriate medication for Andrew to help stem this psychotic episode. His nurse let me know that he had a history of refusing all medications and interventions while hospitalized. He would instead use his time in the psych ward as a sort of "holiday" from the streets. "Three hots and a cot" is an often-used phrase for the stay in the psych ward, just as it is with incarceration.

To be honest, the differentiation between jail and the psychiatric ward is hard to decipher, with the locked doors, bare rooms, contraband items, and unstable inmates. After my initial stint in the psych ward with Andrew, I continued to admit patients there on occasion, but my enthusiasm for work on the psych ward was definitely tempered by my first experience with Andrew.

Chapter 23
Hidden Problem

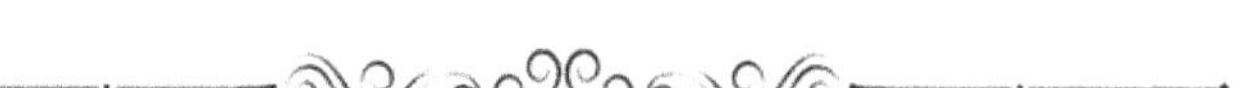

My next interesting case also occurred while I was assigned to work in the Intensive Care Unit.

I was sitting at the nurses' station in the ICU when my pager went off, indicating a new admission from the emergency room. As there wasn't any pressing work for me to do in the ICU at that moment, I decided to go to the ER myself and meet my next admission. Before I left the ICU, I logged on to the computer and looked at my new patient's labs and notes from the ER physicians.

I learned my next patient's name was Cassie, a 20-year-old college student, home on a break from school due to her illness. Cassie had been very ill for the last week, with vomiting and diarrhea. Her symptoms progressed to the point that her family brought her to the hospital. In the ER, she was found to have a high fever of 103, low blood pressure, and a red rash on her body; the classic triad of sepsis. After learning all of the above, I decided it was time to meet her myself.

I entered the mayhem of the ER and marveled at how busy and seemingly chaotic the area appeared, no matter the time of day. I had come to admire the physicians who can work and thrive in such an environment. I found my patient and entered her room. There, she was lying on a stretcher, flanked by her parents. I introduced myself to all three and sat in a chair next to Cassie. She certainly looked uncomfortable, and witnessing her rash and blood pressure of 90/50, I was quite concerned.

After a brief conversation with Cassie and her parents, I decided to find the ER doctor who had been working with her. I needed to know what they were thinking about a diagnosis, and to what ends they had already begun a workup or treatment plan for her. I scoured the area and eventually found Cassie's attending, Dr. ER, coming out of another room.

"Hi, Dr. ER, I'm Dr. Casper. I will be admitting Cassie to the ICU. Can you tell me what you are thinking about her?" I asked him.

"Hi, Dr. Casper, Cassie is not doing well, which is why we are sending her directly to the ICU. Everything in her presentation smells like sepsis, but I haven't been able to locate the source of her infection," he replied. "I'm going to move her upstairs soon. I've already called for transportation."

I decided to go back to the ICU and wait for Cassie, as the ER was packed and I couldn't find anywhere to do my work. Once back in the ICU, I took the opportunity to do some research on sepsis and learned a lot. If Cassie did indeed have sepsis, we would be racing against time to clear her infection before any number of really bad things could happen to her. Sepsis, a blood infection with bacteria, viruses, or fungi, can lead to rapid organ failure and even death if not caught in time and treated appropriately. I was hopeful that I could help unravel the mystery and nidus of her presumed infection.

When Cassie and her parents arrived in the ICU, Cassie was alert and mentating appropriately, but her vital signs were very worrisome, monitored minute by minute on the numerous modalities in the ICU. I entered her room and began my interview with Cassie. She was a typical 20-year-old who attended college in a neighboring state. While there, she became ill and decided to go home to be with her parents. They had been to urgent care twice, where Cassie was given mild antibiotics for a presumed, but not confirmed, urinary tract infection. Even on the antibiotics, Cassie's condition worsened, causing them to bring her to the ER, now earning her a bed in the ICU.

I asked Cassie a lot of questions about activities that could give her an infection, including a detailed sexual history, which was unremarkable, as she was not sexually active. She had been on birth control pills for years, but decided to go off them a few months before admission. She had had her first period in years over a month ago. Cassie denied any recent injuries, cuts, or bruises. She lived in an apartment on campus with two other healthy women. Her parents were unable to provide any information other than reporting that she had new symptoms of nausea, vomiting, and diarrhea.

I finished up with the interview and left Cassie's room to begin my ICU admission orders. I sat at the desk and tried to figure out what had happened to Cassie. She certainly did meet the criteria for sepsis, with her elevated white count, high fever, rash, and low blood pressure. I knew from the research I had done that the biggest concern was a progression from sepsis to septic shock, which has up to a 50% mortality rate. I knew I, with my arsenal of IV fluids, IV antibiotics, and supplemental oxygen, would do my best for her. I finished up the orders and said good night to Cassie and her parents before I left the ICU and headed for the residents' sleeping quarters.

Once in the doctor's sleeping quarters, I quickly fell into a deep sleep. A few hours later, about midnight, I was awakened by a page from the ICU. The page simply read,

"911," which meant there was an emergency there on the unit. I got out of bed and raced to the ICU, uncertain of which patient there needed me. It didn't take long to learn it was Cassie who was in trouble.

I approached Cassie's ICU room and took note of the scene. Her parents were now standing outside her room, and her mother was crying. Inside the room, Cassie was surrounded by nurses and anyone else who could assist in her care. When the charge nurse saw me, she immediately started to bark orders at me. "Dr. Casper, get the crash cart, it's in the storage room right over there," she said as she pointed to a closet across from Cassie's room. At that same moment, I heard the code being called over the hospital's PA system: "Code blue, to the ICU, code blue to the ICU."

In hospitals, a "code blue" is an emergency signal indicating a patient is experiencing cardiac or respiratory arrest. It triggers a rapid response from a team of healthcare professionals, including doctors, nurses, and respiratory therapists, to provide immediate life-saving measures. The purpose of a code blue is to ensure prompt intervention and improve the patient's chance of survival in critical situations.

Every time there is a code blue called in a hospital, one person, usually a doctor, is always designated to be the leader of the code. And, since I was the first doctor to arrive in the ICU, I became the point person to "run the code," responsible for clear communication and defined roles in the patient's room. This meant that I was also responsible for monitoring Cassie's vital signs and shouting out orders for the team to do. "Normal saline, IV push!" I said loudly. "Push one milligram epinephrine!" and so on. I was grateful at that moment that I had paid such close attention to my Advanced Cardiac Life Support (ACLS) training that was required when I entered residency.

I continued to direct the care team as the situation in Cassie's room became more chaotic and frenetic. A physician colleague friend of mine appeared in the room and took his position at the head of the bed, ready to intubate Cassie on my instruction. The room filled up with a variety of people from all over the hospital, as is usual when a code blue is called. Respiratory therapists, nurses, physicians, and any other number of helpers were there to assist as I gave the orders.

I watched the team nervously as they carried out my orders, always staying in my head one step ahead of the mayhem unfolding before me. It was my job to anticipate any eventuality and be prepared for it. I watched Cassie's blood pressure as it continued to decline, and realized that we were dealing with something *really bad* at that point. When her blood pressure plummeted to 65/35, I ordered her intubation and placed her on a ventilator. I then adjusted her medications and put her on continuous vasopressors and IV fluids to help support her blood pressure.

Once Cassie was eventually stabilized on the ventilator, I exited her room and spoke with her parents. I let them know that she most likely had sepsis from an unknown source, and now it has progressed to septic shock, putting her in grave danger of dying. Her extremely low blood pressure was putting her at risk of organ shutdown. I let them know that I would speak with my boss in the morning and that we would continue our workup to try to identify the source of her infection. Her parents were justifiably terrified, but grateful for the care she was receiving.

The next day on rounds, my attending physician, Dr. Stanford, pimped me mercilessly about Cassie. He stated that her elusive diagnosis was most likely staring us in the face; we've just missed it thus far. I admired his confidence and decided to turn over any stone I could in solving her mystery. The situation was now compromised by the fact that Cassie could no longer speak for herself. I directed my attention to the ER notes and my initial interview with her.

Cassie was not doing well, despite the ventilator, IV fluids, and vasopressors. Her vital signs and organs continued to deteriorate. She was on several antibiotics that did not seem to be working, and despite numerous interventions, we couldn't keep her blood pressure up. *Something, somewhere,* was causing her problem, and I was determined to find it. I kept digging.

A few hours later, while sitting outside her room staring at the monitors, I had an idea. I knew it was going to sound crazy to Dr. Stanford, but I decided to float my hypothesis to him anyway, risking humiliation. I was resolute in my desire to solve Cassie's mystery. I found him in his office working on writing a journal article, ironically about sepsis in the ICU.

"Dr. Stanford, I have a thought about Cassie," I said as I entered the tiny room and sat down on a chair.

"That could be interesting, Casper," he replied with an infrequent smile. "She certainly needs help; I'm afraid she could die soon." This was a rare admission from a man of few words, and he didn't soften the blow. I, too, knew Cassie was in grave danger of dying at that point. Another axiom frequently spoken in hospitals is, "Don't let a patient die on your shift," and I was determined that she would not die while under my care.

"I know it may sound crazy, but I think she needs a pelvic exam," I said with as much confidence as I could muster.

"*A pelvic exam?*" Dr. Stanford asked with a puzzled look on his face. It was clear that he may not have had *any* experience with pelvic exams in the decades since his medical school days. I could certainly understand *why* that might not be what he was expecting to hear.

"Yes, you heard me right, a pelvic exam. That's about the only thing we haven't investigated at this point," I replied. "She said she had a period about a month ago, and hasn't had one since. I didn't get into more detail with her before she was intubated, but I am worried about a retained tampon."

"You sure do come up with some crazy ideas, Casper, but I do see your point," Dr. Stanford stated. "Do you want to do the exam yourself, or call OBGYN?"

"I can do it. I will speak with her parents, obtain their consent, and get the room set up," I finished.

"You go, Casper," Dr. Stanford said and gave me the "thumbs up" sign. He appeared thrilled that I did not ask for his assistance, and he happily went back to his computer work.

I ordered the supplies I would need for the pelvic exam and had Cassie's parents sign the consent. It took several nursing personnel to help me perform the pelvic exam in an ICU bed on a ventilated patient. Before I inserted the speculum, I palpated Cassie's pelvis and thought I felt a small mass behind the uterus. I then inserted the speculum and viewed the problem: Cassie had a retained tampon tucked up behind her uterus, most likely from a month prior, when she had had her menses.

I inserted the forceps into her vagina and pulled out the retained tampon. It was black with infection and smelled like a sewer. It took all my will not to gag at that point. I placed the tampon in a sterile container and sent it to the lab for analysis. I then used normal saline and tried to flush and clean out her vagina as much as I could before ending the procedure. Once done, I went to find Dr. Stanford to report the good news.

"Dr. Stanford, Cassie's problem has been found and dealt with," I said, trying to sound succinct and professional.

"Go on, you didn't," he replied. "What did you find?"

"A retained tampon, probably a month old, and definitely what was causing her problem. I sent it to the lab for a STAT evaluation. Hopefully, we can save her," I replied.

"Strong work, Casper. I like it when you rotate through my ICU," Dr. Stanford replied before he turned his attention back to his article.

I couldn't believe what I was hearing. *"He likes me, he really likes me,"* an old quote from a once-famous actress ran through my head.

I continued to follow Cassie for the remainder of her time in the ICU. She started to improve almost immediately after the tampon and nidus of her infection was removed from her body. Once the pathogen had been identified from the tampon, we were able to tailor her antibiotics to the best one for her problem. Over the ensuing days, she slowly got better and was eventually able to be extubated, and other supportive measures were weaned. Cassie had literally survived septic shock, and we were all so happy for her and her family.

It was "wins" like this, and the ability to actually help someone get better, that keeps you going in medicine. It is a satisfaction that is hard to describe.

Chapter 24
Mr. Fitness

As a medical doctor and senior resident, I eventually came to really like the Intensive Care Unit.

I liked the acuity of the patients and the teamwork of the crew there. The camaraderie of the care team made up for the lack of interaction with my patients. Most in the ICU were unable to communicate with me for one reason or another: intubation, coma, sepsis, etc. Occasionally, we would admit someone to the ICU who was able to fully communicate with us. Midway through my next ICU rotation, one such patient got admitted to my service.

Usually, when a patient gets admitted to the ICU, due to the acuity of the situation, you spend the majority of your time reading copious prior chart notes, if available, and meeting with family members. This next patient, however, was admitted fully awake, alert, and seemingly ready for the necessary medical treatment.

I was sitting at the nurses' station when Mr. Fitness was admitted to the ICU. I saw him out of the corner of my eye as he was wheeled past me, and noticed that he was an unusually good-looking, 65-year-old middle-aged man. He had a deep tan, out of keeping with the cold climate where he was being admitted.

There weren't any chart notes to review on Mr. Fitness because he had never been admitted to our hospital before. Additionally, he had rarely seen a doctor in his life as he was exceedingly healthy before this admission. Upon presentation to our hospital, he was so sick that he had been admitted directly to the ICU from the ER. This usually means something really bad is going on. I had been told by the ER attending that Mr. Fitness would need emergent dialysis for acute kidney failure. This was the reason for his ICU admission, as dialysis could be performed at the bedside there.

Although ostensibly being admitted to the ICU for hemodialysis, I had to admit, Mr. Fitness didn't look very sick at all, in comparison to other patients on the unit. He was incredibly handsome and fit for his age, and shared with me that he was an avid rock climber. He was married with three grown daughters, four grandchildren, and had retired from a very successful career in aerospace. Until recently, he took no medications and had avoided doctors for most of his life.

A month before his admission, at a rare doctor appointment, his primary care physician had put him on an angiotensin converting enzyme (ACE) inhibitor for extremely mild hypertension. There is a standard of care with the initiation of this medicine, requiring the physician to check the patient's kidney function both *before* starting the drug and a week later. This is done to make sure that everything is okay with the patient's kidneys. Specifically, you must check and monitor the patient's blood urea nitrogen (BUN) and creatinine, two markers of kidney health.

Mr. Fitness's primary care doctor had failed to perform either blood test on him when he initiated the antihypertensive drug. Over the previous month, Mr. Fitness was blissfully unaware that something devastating was going on in his body. At the time of admission, he had just returned from a week of intensive rock climbing, where he had begun to feel unwell.

While camping and in relative wilderness, Mr. Fitness had experienced extreme fatigue, nausea, shortness of breath, brown urine, and a significant swelling of his lower legs. He cut his trip short due to these symptoms and presented to the ER. Upon admission, he had a BUN/Creatinine ratio of 100/10, respectively, indicating severe, acute kidney failure. That was the highest BUN/Creatinine ratio that I had ever seen.

Kidney failure occurs when the kidneys lose their ability to filter waste products and excess fluids from the blood. It can be acute, as in Mr. Fitness's case, caused by a pharmaceutical drug or some other insult. Or, it can be chronic, developing over many years from a variety of causes. Mr. Fitness exhibited all of the classic signs of acute kidney failure with his leg swelling, fatigue, weakness, and dark urine. Treatment includes stopping the offending drug, which we did, and emergent hemodialysis.

Dialysis is required when your kidneys can no longer filter toxins and waste products from the blood into your urine. Once commenced, dialysis is usually permanent, but not always. Hemodialysis is a procedure where the cleaning of your blood is done with a dialysis machine external to the body. Your blood circulates out of your body to a "cleaning machine," then the filtered blood is reintroduced back into your body.

Dialysis is a complex procedure used for kidney failure, and is rarely temporary. Once commenced, dialysis patients are usually committed for the rest of their lives to thrice-weekly, multi-hour dialysis sessions at one of the ubiquitous "dialysis centers." Due to the acute and recent injury to his kidneys, we were pretty confident that Mr. Fitness's dialysis would be temporary, once his kidneys were given the chance to recover.

I spent quite a bit of time with Mr. Fitness and had an initial conversation with him about dialysis. I let him know that, although unusual, his hemodialysis needs were most likely a transient measure. I shared that he could quite possibly return to having normally functioning kidneys after we gave them a little break with hemodialysis. He might need dialysis for no more than a week or two, the ICU team and I thought. He asked me lots of questions about dialysis, and I did my best to give him accurate information, fully aware of my knowledge limitations.

Throughout our initial conversation, I never thought that Mr. Fitness would consider dialysis to be an *option*, given that there really wasn't another choice to restore him to good health. So, I spoke with him as though this invasive medical intervention was a fait accompli. But as our initial time together progressed, I eventually realized that he wasn't asking me questions to understand *what* he was about to go through, but rather to decide *if* he would go through with dialysis.

"Mr. Fitness, do you have any more questions for me before I get you set up for dialysis?" I asked at the conclusion of our interview and exam.

"Yes, tell me *why* I should go through with this dialysis," he replied.

"Why?" I asked in disbelief, trying to maintain a poker face. "Well, it will most likely be temporary, just enough time for your kidneys to recover from the insult from the ACE inhibitor. Our goal from dialysis is to restore you to good health again."

"But, you can't say that's for sure, right?" he asked.

"Correct. But without dialysis, you won't survive," I replied, feeling instantly like a jerk for saying so, but he did seem like a no-nonsense kind of guy.

"At this point, I'm going to decline," Mr. Fitness finished.

I couldn't believe what I was hearing. *Decline dialysis? Decline living? Decline seeing your grandchildren grow up?*

I wasn't sure how to respond at that point and took my time as I thought carefully of what to say next. "Mr. Fitness, why don't I come back and meet with you again once your wife and family get here?" I suggested.

"That won't be necessary," he replied. "They will respect my wishes."

"Mr. Fitness, we didn't discuss this, but are you depressed?" I asked as I sat back down on the bedside chair.

"Not at all. I've had an amazing life full of adventure and happiness. At this point, I am competent to make my own decisions," he replied. "If it's my time to go, then so be it," he stated.

I was speechless at that point as I did not expect that reply from him at all. "Mr. Fitness, I will have your nurse page me when your family arrives. Please reconsider your decision," I said as I stood up, gently grabbed his hand in mine, and gave him a warm smile. "I am sure your family will want you to stay around a little longer," I finished and walked out of the room with tears in my eyes.

I made it a point to find Dr. Stanford right away to let him know what had transpired with Mr. Fitness. He was as shocked as I was with the current state of affairs with him. He suggested that we get an emergency Ethics Committee Consultation to see if we could compel Mr. Fitness to accept dialysis. A full consultation was not necessary as I got all the information I needed by simply stopping by their office. The ethics team let me know that the law was quite clear: If Mr. Fitness is competent, anything short of honoring his decisions, no matter how much we - or anyone - disagreed with him, would amount to legal battery. We could not compel him to receive treatment and choose life.

I spent the next 48 hours meeting extensively with Mr. Fitness and his family, some of the nicest people I have ever met. While no one in his family wanted him to die, and certainly not at that time in his life, they all respected his autonomy and ability to make his own decisions.

Mr. Fitness remained steadfast in his refusal to accept any intervention, despite his kidney situation most likely being temporary and reversible. Dr. Stanford had also made him aware of the fact that his illness was a result of medical malpractice. Despite all this, Mr. Fitness was undeterred in his decision to reject any treatment.

Death from kidney failure is actually a pretty good way to go. When your kidneys can't do their work, the buildup of toxins in the blood, as the body shuts down, allows the patient to be quite comfortable, and a bit "high." Mr. Fitness didn't last much longer after his admission to the ICU, and we decided as a team to let him stay there, rather than transferring him out to the busy and chaotic wards. Moving a patient around the hospital can be quite disruptive, and we wanted to make his remaining time on earth as smooth as possible for his family and him.

We asked Hospice to get involved, and they provided much comfort to his family. Mr. Fitness passed away peacefully with a smile on his face, with his wife, daughters, and me at his bedside. Once again, Dr. Death was at her patient's side as they transitioned. After pronouncing him dead, I sat at the nurses' station with tears streaming down my face as his family stayed with him and surrounded his bed.

I was so grateful that I was able to be with him as he moved from his amazing life here on earth to hopefully an even better place elsewhere, where he could climb rocks with abandon.

Chapter 25
Devil in the Details

Toward the end of my time in residency, I had one remaining month on the internal medicine wards. Patients on these units had innumerable different diagnoses like pneumonia, cancer, gall bladder problems, pulmonary embolisms, kidney infections, and so on. To earn a bed in our busy hospital, you really had to be pretty sick. Mrs. Mark was one such patient.

"Hey Doc," my attending physician said playfully as I passed him in the hall one morning. "I'd like you to pick up our new admission, Mrs. Mark. She is not doing well in our institution, and I am hoping you can figure out why. She has become a true medical mystery. I heard through the hospital grapevine that you actually like these vexing cases. If you can't figure out what's going on with her, she is headed for Hospice," he finished with his thinly veiled threat.

I already had a full service and didn't relish another patient on my census, especially a complex one who was a medical mystery. I guess a bit of "senioritis" had started to set in. "No problem," I replied cheerily as I smiled at him. "I'll go see her now."

Mrs. Mark was assigned to me as a "new" admission to my ward service, but she had been in our hospital for over a month. She was 78 years old with multiple medical problems. Initially, she was admitted for worsening heart failure and a urinary tract infection. And at first, she had improved with antibiotics, and after Lasix took ten pounds of water off of her. But, after that initial improvement, Mrs. Mark had had a steady deterioration ever since. Her heart rate had consistently declined over the past few weeks, and now it was my job to try and figure out why.

I was admitting Mrs. Mark to the internal medicine wards as a transfer from the Cardiac Care Unit (CCU), rather than through the emergency department. She had initially been admitted to the Intensive Care Unit, where she was stabilized with Lasix and antibiotics before she was transferred to the wards (a step down). While on the wards, she did not do well, so a week later, Mrs. Mark was transferred from the wards to the CCU due to her ever-slowing heart rate. She stayed in the CCU for a week, but the cause of her bradycardia was not discovered by the CCU team.

Mrs. Mark's advanced directive status was Do Not Resuscitate (DNR), so her family had decided against the placement of a pacemaker. At that point, the decision was made to transfer her from the CCU back to the wards, assuming that she would ultimately not survive this hospitalization. This is where and when I began to care for her.

Despite all of the time in the hospital and the multiple medical interventions she received, Mrs. Mark had continued to decline under our care. Of greatest concern was her declining heart rate, 27 beats per minute when I met her. As usual, I familiarized myself with Mrs. Mark's chart and lab results before I met her. She indeed was a vexing internal medicine case, and I had inches of paperwork to review just from her time in our institution alone.

At the time that I met Mrs. Mark, computerized orders were not available in hospitals yet, and most communication between providers, ancillary hospital staff, and pharmacists was done with pen, paper, and carbon copies. As was standard practice at that time in our hospital, each time a patient was moved from one floor or care unit to another, a completely new set of orders had to be handwritten in the patient's paper chart. This meant rewriting the entire long list of medications she was on.

Mrs. Mark was on multiple medications, including an ACE inhibitor and hydrochlorothiazide for her hypertension. She was also on Coumadin for atrial fibrillation, digoxin for heart failure, a statin for cholesterol, metformin for diabetes, and, not surprisingly, an SSRI for depression. Her daily cocktail of medications was impressive, and had been handwritten and rewritten several times during her hospitalization with us thus far.

I studied her chart and multiple orders from a plethora of physicians, attempting to find a cause for her failing health. At that time, all patient orders were handwritten in paper charts. After each medication ordered was written by a physician, a carbon copy of that order was physically sent to the pharmacy, where a pharmacist once again transcribed the doctor's order for said medication. Then, and only then, was medication dispensed to the patient.

It didn't matter if the patient was on one medication or twenty-one; the medications and dosages were written, rewritten, and double checked at several different points before being dispensed to a patient. Thankfully, medication errors in our hospital were rare.

I started my detective work with her original admission orders, now about one month old. I reviewed all of her medications ordered and compared the list to the one she provided from her care home, where she resided. All seemed copacetic. Nothing initially stood out to me as something I could fix. I decided to go meet my new patient. I entered Mrs. Mark's room and introduced myself to her after I found the TV remote and turned off the blaring TV playing a game show. She was an attractive elderly woman who looked her age, but somewhat frail.

"Hello, Mrs. Mark, I'm Dr. Casper," I said as I pulled up a chair to sit beside her bed.

"*Another* doctor?" she replied with a sigh. "I haven't met you before."

"I know. You're probably getting sick of us doctors by now. I know I would be," I replied, trying to show empathy for what she had been through. "I am here to see if we can *finally* figure out why your heart rate is so low."

"You would think *someone* would know what's going on with me," she shot back.

"Well, hopefully we will get this figured out soon," I finished.

I spent quite a bit of time performing Mrs. Mark's physical exam, emphasizing her cardiac exam. I couldn't find anything out of the ordinary except her heart rate of 27 beats per minute. Her heart rate was nearly equal to her respiration rate. I had never met someone with such a low heart rate, and I was impressed that she was mentating so well.

"Well, Mrs. Mark, I'm going to discuss your care with my supervisor. Please don't lose hope. I know I haven't lost hope," I finished. I tucked her back underneath the sheet and turned the television back on before leaving her room.

I decided against looking for my boss as I really didn't have anything intelligent to report to him. Instead, I sat back down at the nurses' station and pulled out Mrs. Mark's huge chart again. I couldn't shake the feeling that her chart held the secret to her declining health. *Something, somewhere, somehow* in her thick chart should reveal itself to me. If only I tried harder, I told myself.

After helping myself to a cup of lukewarm coffee from the ward's kitchen, I pored over her chart. I lost track of time and missed my children's dinner and bedtimes. I was resolute that Mrs. Mark would not be placed in Hospice care if I had anything to do with it.

Bradycardia, or a slow heart rate, is sometimes not a cause for concern. Elite athletes generally have slow heart rates, often less than 60 beats per minute, indicating exceptional health. But bradycardia in the elderly is never a good sign, and usually an indicator of a sick heart. Mrs. Mark did indeed have an ailing heart, but bradycardia was a *new* problem for her since the time of admission to our hospital a month earlier. I decided to turn my attention to her extensive medication list.

Mrs. Mark was on a medication called digoxin for her heart failure. Digoxin's purpose is to regulate the heart rate and help an ill or failing heart to contract better. As a therapy, digoxin is a double-edged sword as it has a very narrow therapeutic window. Meaning, the dosing is strict and tightly regulated by taking frequent blood levels of the drug. The usual and highest dose, and the dose Mrs. Mark was on at home, was 0.25 milligrams daily. When I had admitted her to my service earlier in the day, I had written for that same amount of digoxin, the standard of care.

I scoured Mrs. Mark's history in the hospital, looking specifically at her medication orders. I started with her admission through the emergency room a month earlier. I checked the medication list and noticed an error: the admitting physician had ordered 2.5 mg of digoxin for her rather than 0.25 mg. This was a tenfold increase from her prescribed dose. One tiny error of one decimal point that over time had had a devastating, overdose impact on her.

That same medication error had followed her throughout her hospital stay on multiple different wards, multiple different physicians, and multiple different pharmacies within the hospital. I had completely missed the errors the first time I reviewed her chart earlier that day, simply ordering the correct dose when I wrote her new admission orders.

Digoxin overdose causes bradycardia, and if unchecked, it can be fatal. Once I found the error - and the iatrogenic cause of her problem - I paged my attending supervisor. He was eating in the Doctor's Dining Room and invited me to join him. I happily did so as I hadn't had a chance to eat all day.

I grabbed a little dinner from the aging buffet and sat down next to my boss. I was grateful to find that at that late hour, we were alone in the dining room. I didn't want to be overheard as I gave him the news. I ate a few bites of my dinner before revealing the mystery of Mrs. Mark.

"Well, Dr. Casey, I found the problem with Mrs. Mark," I offered.

"You're not serious! Already?" he replied as he gave me a high-five salute and a smile. "So, no Hospice for her? Tell me more."

"Dr. Casey, I'm actually kind of embarrassed to tell you the problem," I started.

"Embarrassed, detective? Why is that?" he asked in reply with a puzzled look on his face.

"Well, *we* caused her bradycardia," I stated.

"Tell me more, Einstein," he said as he continued to eat.

"Well, ever since her time of admission about a month ago, she's been receiving 2.5 mg of digoxin daily," I said. "That first erroneous order was written by the physician in the ER and has followed her ever since," I continued.

"Excuse me? Did you say 2.5 mg? Ten times the upper limit?" That's a toxic dose of digoxin!" he replied in disbelief.

"Yes, you heard me right, and she's been receiving that dose for a month. Her medication orders have been rewritten in this hospital several times over the past month. Each time, the digoxin order was written for 2.5 mg, and quite surprisingly, each of the pharmacies in our hospital actually dispensed it to her."

"Holy crap!" he said excitedly and paused his eating. "First of all, nice work, Detective Casper. Second, you will need to present her case to the hospital's Morbidity & Mortality Committee meeting next week. I am the chair of the committee and will put you on the agenda. This obviously shouldn't have happened," he finished as he turned his attention back to his dinner.

We finished our meal in silence before I returned to the wards to finish up for the day. Before I left the hospital for the night, I wrote an order in Mrs. Mark's chart to immediately discontinue her digoxin.

It is estimated that approximately 440,000 people die or are seriously injured in the U.S. every year due to medical errors, also called iatrogenic errors. Meaning, the error was caused by the medical system itself. Medication errors in hospitals make up 52% of the errors experienced and are a significant patient safety concern. This contributes to adverse drug events, prolonged hospital stays, and increased healthcare costs.

Medication errors are found as prescribing errors, as in this case; administration errors, as in this case; dispensing errors, as in this case; and monitoring errors. Mrs. Mark could have had a digoxin level monitored at any time over the previous month, which would have shown the toxic level in her blood. But as the medication error was not in their differential diagnosis of her bradycardia, no one on the staff had thought to check a digoxin level.

Studies have shown that medication errors in hospitals occur 5-10% of the time globally. Even more concerning, a 2018 *British Medical Journal* study found error rates as high as 20% in some hospital settings. Errors are found particularly in the ICUs, where copious different drugs are ordered for most patients. Adverse drug events (ADEs) range from mild, like a rash, to severe, where you can see organ failure or death. Errors in medication dispensing also increase the length of hospital stays and litigation expenses. This is estimated to cost between $20-40 billion dollars annually in the U.S.

In situations like what happened with Mrs. Mark, physicians must decide whether and how to disclose medical mistakes, balancing honesty with potential legal or professional repercussions. A recent study showed that what patients want most, after a medical error has occurred, is transparency and an apology from the medical establishment. Regardless, patients receive disclosure less than 30% of the time after a medical error or mistake has occurred.

Before I left the hospital for the day, I decided to give Mrs. Mark the "good" news. I let her know we were adjusting one of her medications and that she should start to feel better very soon. This was a true story, but not the *whole truth*. In this case with Mrs. Mark, the decision was made by the team to not disclose the medication mistake.

It took about a week for her system to flush out the toxic level of digoxin, and she was ultimately able to be discharged back to her care home with a normal heart rate.

Interlogue
Introduction to Medical Practice

The graduation from internship and residency is a milestone that doctors wait years, if not over a decade, for, depending on the specialty they choose. Graduation ceremonies are celebratory and filled with hope and promise for your future. By this time, most physicians in training have secured a "real job," and often consider this graduation rite of passage the final steppingstone to completing a life goal. At this time in your medical training, you are expected to employ in your chosen specialty a combination of scientific knowledge, clinical skills, and patient-centered care.

As a newly minted, full-fledged doctor, you no longer have attendings to guide, shape, and nurture your learning. But likewise, no more attendings to haze, criticize, or mistreat you. You've reached your sometimes life-long goal and are ready to be released into the world of medicine as a fully-trained doctor. You are assumed to be prepared to diagnose, treat, and prevent illnesses and injuries.

But the learning process doesn't end at graduation. It actually becomes more acute when you are now the "top dog" in the medical hierarchy. Fortunately, medicine eventually kept pace with technology, and at the time of my graduation from residency, there were comprehensive websites dedicated to the practice of medicine, aiding in my ability to provide appropriate care to my patients.

Medical school and residency had trained me well, and I was grateful for the incredible learning opportunities I had had over the previous decade. After considering several different career options, I decided to look for employment as a physician in an outpatient clinic setting.

Upon graduation from residency, I fell into a coveted private practice job in a beautiful outpatient setting. The hours were long, and the patients were sometimes vexing or difficult. But the sense of accomplishment in surviving medical training usually kept me energetic and optimistic.

The following are a few stories from my time in private practice.

Chapter 26
Ethics in the Operating Room

After graduating from my residency, I worked as a private practice physician in my hometown. Suddenly, I was not only a full-fledged doctor, but I was now an employer of my team of ancillary medical providers and support staff. I found the work to be highly rewarding, but somewhat isolating from other physicians.

I missed my days in the hospital where colleagues of all specialties collaborate via "curbside consultations," and commune casually in places like the doctor's dining room. I even missed the bad coffee, graham crackers, and peanut butter from the nurse's station. I decided it was time to network with other outpatient, clinic-based physicians in my community.

As a female physician and specialist, I was asked nearly daily - mostly by my female patients - for a recommendation to a plastic surgeon for a variety of concerns. I felt it was my duty to "screen" my colleagues for the best person to refer to, as my referral to another physician could ultimately reflect on me. I only wanted the best for my patients, no matter who was providing their care, or for what concern.

I decided one day to reach out to a plastic surgery colleague to foster a relationship of referrals. I set my sights on one particular plastic surgeon, whom I had met previously at a medical meeting. He was a respected doctor in his specialty. His office was close to mine, and he seemed like a good fit for my plastic surgery referrals. I was excited at the thought of establishing a collegial relationship with him.

Dr. Plastic was tall, fit, extremely handsome, arrogant, and, according to my assessment of his results, highly competent. He had a reputation in town of being the best aesthetic plastic surgeon, although the most expensive. Most patients were willing to pay his exorbitant fees for his exceptional results. He was a "big fish" in our city's pond, and he seemed to be a perfect fit for my patient referrals. Slightly intimidated, I placed a call to his office to set up an appointment to meet him. I wanted to discuss with him how he would handle the patients that I would send to him for surgery.

Dr. Plastic invited me to his beautiful office building, which he owned. There, he had a medical spa and a fully-accredited operating room of his own. On our tour, I was impressed with both his beautiful staff and him. His gorgeous wife was his office manager, something that was quite common at that time, and they made a formidable pair. We finished our office tour by convening in his conference room.

"Beautiful office, Dr. Plastic," I said as we sat down. I could see why his patients loved coming to see him.

"Thank you, Liz," he replied, eliminating the formality of "doctor." I was too intimidated to call him by his first name.

"Thank you for agreeing to see my patient referrals," I stated. "I do have one request."

"What's that, Liz?" he replied, looking surprised.

"If I send you a patient whom you plan to provide plastic surgery to, I would like to join you for the surgery," I answered. I knew this was an unconventional request, but I wanted to see *how* he achieved his near-perfect results. He agreed without hesitation, and I was excited at the budding professional relationship I felt was forming. After a short while together, Dr. Plastic indicated he had to go and see a patient, so I left and returned to my own office to see my patients.

It didn't take long after my visit to Dr. Plastic before another female patient asked me for a referral to a plastic surgeon. This patient, Mrs. Wood, was a 75-year-old woman who wanted to see an aesthetic plastic surgeon for an upper and lower blepharoplasty. This procedure, commonly called an eyelid lift, improves the appearance of the eyes by removing excess fat and/or skin. Done wrong or poorly, surgery on the eyes can completely change a person's appearance, and not always for the better. Dr. Plastic had the reputation of being the best aesthetic surgeon in our city for this delicate procedure on the eyes.

Mrs. Wood had the typical appearance of someone her age who had neglected her appearance for decades, and it showed. Overweight, with saggy jowls, multiple chins, midface drooping, bags under her eyes, and heavy eyelids. But she herself was only concerned about her eyes.

Mrs. Wood wanted to get the surgery done as soon as possible before her upcoming college reunion. She needed time to both get the procedure and to heal before the event. She let me know she was on a very tight budget and, although she would like to "do more" surgically, getting her eyes done was all she could afford at that time.

I called Dr. Plastic while Mrs. Wood was still in my office. I told him about the desired blepharoplasty, and he agreed to see her right away, rather than the usual three-month wait for an appointment to be seen with him. He said he would let me know the date and time of her surgery so that I could schedule accordingly to join him for the procedure. A week or so later, Dr. Plastic's wife called me to inform me of the date of Mrs. Wood's planned surgery, and I adjusted my own schedule so that I could join them.

On the morning of the surgery, I put on my own scrubs and drove to Dr. Plastic's office at 7:30 a.m. As I entered the waiting room, I said hello to Mrs. Wood and let her know I would be joining her for the surgery. She thanked me profusely for being there and appeared very excited about the surgery on her eyes. I gave her a brief hug and exited the waiting room through a door labeled "private."

I met with Dr. Plastic briefly in his office before we scrubbed in together at the sink located outside his operating room. We didn't discuss the surgery he had planned for Mrs. Wood, and I assumed it was a blepharoplasty. Instead, we discussed current events and sports scores. We learned that our children attended school in the same school district, and Dr. Plastic even suggested we get our families together for a barbecue at his home at some future point. I was feeling very comfortable and pleased with my decision to refer patients to him.

After we scrubbed in, we entered the OR together and donned our sterile gowns, masks, and gloves. By that time, Mrs. Wood was resting on the operating table and getting prepped and anesthetized for the surgery by a team of nurses. Dr. Plastic took his seat at the head of the table, and I took a seat on the opposite side of Mrs. Wood's head. Dr.

Plastic asked for his favorite music to be played, and he began the operation once Mrs. Wood was fully asleep.

Instead of approaching the eyes, Dr. Plastic placed his scalpel at the front of her ear and began to cut. Although I myself was far from being a plastic surgeon, I knew enough about facial plastic surgery to know he was not intending to work on her eyes at that moment. I stayed quiet and did not ask any questions, remembering my time in the OR as a student and resident.

Instead, I watched his every move as he carefully and expertly lifted the tissues of her neck, her midface, *and* her upper face. It was a massive surgery for someone her age, encompassing her whole face, with prolonged anesthesia.

I sat motionless and silent for the four-hour procedure, watching as Dr. Plastic lifted her entire face, a procedure that would typically cost $25,000 with this surgeon. I remembered Mrs. Wood's assertion that she could only afford to have her eyes addressed. After stapling her face and neck tissues back together in their new place, he draped her entire head and scalp in the typical bandages seen after a facelift procedure. I assumed he was saving her eyes for last. The piece de resistance, if you will. Boy, was I misguided.

"Well, Dr. Casper," he said in front of his nursing staff, "we are done here." He stood over the patient and took off his gloves, mask, and gown, breaking the sterile field and confirming the operation was over. I looked at him with a quizzical look, then back at the patient. I was confused about the lack of surgery on her eyes, the only thing she wanted, or could afford to fix.

I began to feel like a medical student, back in the OR with an intimidating attending, even though he and I were now colleagues. I wasn't sure if I should say something. I decided I had nothing to lose; after all, Mrs. Wood was only *in* his OR because of *my* referral to him. I felt he owed me an explanation at that point.

"What about her eyes, Dr. Plastic, the reason she came to see you?" I asked in earnest, hoping I wasn't stepping on his toes.

He bent toward me over a still-sleeping Mrs. Wood and looked directly at me. He said in a hushed tone, "Don't worry, she'll be back! I'll let you know when she schedules her eyes."

I couldn't believe what I was hearing. Mrs. Wood now likely had a $25,000 bill, and her eyes still looked terrible, made more so by the adjacent surgery on the other parts of her face. I wondered how and why she had ended up with this surgical plan. I also wondered if she was even aware that her eyes would not be addressed after such an extensive and expensive surgery.

Dr. Plastic's nurses began to prepare to move Mrs. Wood to the recovery area, and it was clear the operation was over. I stood up, took off my sterile garb, and exited the OR. Dr. Plastic immediately began to dictate the procedure into a hand-held Dictaphone as he headed back to his office. We didn't debrief after the surgery, and I had to head back to my own office and patients before Mrs. Wood awakened from the anesthesia.

This was the first - and only time - I referred any patients to Dr. Plastic.

Chapter 27
Cherie

Cherie was one of my favorite patients. She came from a distant small town to see me for her specialty care in the city.

I had been in private practice for several years when I met Cherie for the first time. I saw her yearly, if not more frequently, for issues related to my medical expertise. She was middle-aged, overweight, with a BMI of 29, and had somewhat masculine features. She was happily married with three grown children.

Over the years, Cherie began to share with me symptoms she was experiencing, including new-onset headaches, which is never a good sign. I urged her to see a neurologist, which she eventually did. But she reported to me that the referral process from her primary care physician took months for her to even schedule an appointment.

The next time I saw Cherie in my office, about a year later, she reported that the community neurologist had essentially blown her off. He blamed the headaches on her sedentary lifestyle and overweight BMI. He also didn't order any imaging studies. At this visit with me, Cherie reported a worsening of her headaches and also reported that she was having trouble with her teeth. Both of these topics were outside of my purview as her physician. I encouraged her to see her primary care physician again, and also her dentist, to investigate the problem with her teeth.

About another year later, I saw Cherie again, and her appearance took me by surprise. Never what you could call very attractive, Cherie's face now seemed to be a bit more masculine. She had more pronounced features, including a stronger brow and chin. She now reported needing to buy larger shoes as her feet were growing bigger despite no weight gain. This new symptom, in addition to her other reports of problems with headaches, her changing appearance, and her teeth, gave me pause.

Perhaps it's time for this detective to go to work? I asked myself, thinking of all the medical mysteries I had participated in during medical school and residency. At this point, obscure diagnoses started to emerge from the recesses of my mind and distant medical training. Always taught to look for horses (or common diagnoses), I was now a sleuth looking for the medical zebra.

Something was certainly going on with Cherie, but no one thus far had figured it out. Other physicians she had seen seemed to be content with the lack of a definitive diagnosis. Instead, electing to leave her to suffer with progressing and changing symptoms. I also realized at that point that I was more worried about her symptoms than she was. I didn't want to scare her, but I felt the need to help her further if I could.

I sat down next to Cherie and asked to see her hands. As she stretched out her arms toward me to reveal her hands, I was taken aback. Gone was her beautiful wedding ring, which I had so often admired. "Cherie, where is your wedding ring?" I asked, concerned for her marriage.

"I had to have my ring cut off because my hands have grown so much," she replied. I reached out to hold and examine her hands and was struck by how large they were. Almost like baseball mitts, and devoid of any feminine features.

"How long have your hands and feet been growing?" I asked as I started to formulate a differential diagnosis list in my mind.

Simultaneously, my nurse knocked on my exam room door to let me know that my next patient was ready and waiting for me. Cherie's diagnosis detour, not even in my area of practice in medicine, could totally derail my morning's schedule. But, at that point, I felt it was too important to leave her hanging and let her leave my office. Her primary care physician, her neurologist, and her dentist had all failed Cherie. I decided to delay seeing my next patient to investigate further.

"Cherie, I'd like to examine your mouth, if you don't mind," I stated.

"Of course, but my dentist wasn't concerned," she offered.

"I understand, but I want to see for myself. I have a hunch," I replied.

Cherie moved from a chair to the examination table. I took the otoscope from the wall unit and moved the light to her open mouth. I picked up a tongue blade to move her tongue, but I really didn't need to use it. I shined the light on the top of her mouth and was shocked to see another partial set of teeth. They were protruding from the roof of her mouth, mirroring the shape of her permanent teeth. "Cherie, are you aware of these extra teeth?" I asked.

"Yes, they've been there for years, but lately they seem to be growing in size and number," she replied.

"What did your dentist say about these extra teeth?" I asked, trying not to sound horrified or judgmental.

"My dentist said this can happen as we age, and he wasn't worried," she replied.

"Interesting," I said, trying to contain my growing rage. A working diagnosis had formed in my mind. *Were her other physicians really unable to put this puzzle together?*

I asked Cherie to once again sit next to me on a chair. "Cherie, I know you are not here to see me for these worsening symptoms. But I hope you will allow me to give my opinion. I care about you," I said earnestly.

"Of course, I trust you implicitly. And to be honest, no one else has taken me seriously or been able to help me," she replied. "I kind of feel like you are my only lifeline."

"I know it's going to sound crazy, but I believe you could have a tumor in the part of your brain that controls such things as growth hormone. Normally, growth hormone is tightly regulated and tapers off as we age. Growth hormone allows you to grow from an infant to an adult. Rarely, actually very rarely, there can be abnormal growth in an area of the brain called the pituitary gland. This is the gland that regulates this critical hormone. Most often, these tumors are benign, but brain surgery is usually required. But surgery is highly effective for treating this problem," I finished.

At this point, my nurse was knocking on the door again, and tears were welling up in Cherie's eyes.

"A freaking brain tumor?" she implored. "How on earth did you think of *that*?" she continued. I knew her fear, disbelief, and anger were not directed at me. I was simply the messenger of a diagnosis no one wants to receive.

"I'm so sorry, but the good news is that if I'm right, you should begin to feel better after surgery. My working diagnosis of acromegaly - which must be confirmed by a neurosurgeon - was made by linking up all of your seemingly disparate symptoms. I've had the good fortune of seeing you over the years and have been able to see the progression of your symptoms. Think of me as your medical detective with a holistic view of your health," I replied. "I'm looking at you from a 30,000-foot view. It gives me a different perspective."

"Each time I've seen you over the years, you have had consistent complaints that continue to grow: headaches, teeth problems, and growing hands and feet. This all leads me to a probable diagnosis of a medical zebra: a pituitary tumor. Unfortunately, many of your symptoms will not improve or regress after surgery, but your headaches should fully resolve. The changes in your hands, feet, face, and teeth are unfortunately permanent. It is good to catch this tumor now, before any other irreversible changes occur," I finished.

A pituitary adenoma is a benign, non-cancerous tumor that develops in this small gland, located deep in the base of the brain. It regulates hormones, such as growth hormone, as seen in Cheri's case. The incidence of these tumors in the general population is 10-20%. And some are found as an incidental finding, with few or no clinical sequelae. The tumors are graded on both size and function. Left untreated, pituitary tumors may lead to permanent vision loss, hormone imbalances, or, rarely, bleeding into the tumor.

Excess growth hormone from a pituitary adenoma can have a wide range of symptoms and effects. This depends on the age of the individual when the excess growth hormone occurs. If growth hormone is found in excess during childhood or adolescence, gigantism can occur, leading to abnormal height and body size (think seven feet tall with a large head, hands, and feet).

You can also see some of the same sequelae when excess growth hormone occurs in an adult: enlarged hands and feet; coarse, masculine facial features; excess teeth; headaches; and more. Adults with growth hormone overgrowth, called acromegaly, do not get taller, but do experience all of the other side effects.

Before she left the office, I gave Cherie the names of a couple of really good neurosurgeons in town. She would need to get a proper referral from her primary care doctor. I saw her about six months after her successful surgery for a benign pituitary adenoma, and she was doing well. Her headaches had completely resolved, and she had had her wedding ring resized to fit her new hands.

While she continued to credit me with her diagnosis, I was forever grateful to the neurosurgeon who ultimately cured her.

Chapter 28
Adventures in Flying

Part of being a physician includes taking classes every year to maintain your knowledge through courses called "CME," or Continuing Medical Education. Early in my career, online CME courses really weren't available, so traveling to take these courses was commonplace and expected.

One such CME course in my specialty was being held in Las Vegas at a time and date I could attend. I adjusted my clinic schedule and booked a ticket on Southwest Airlines.

The morning of the flight to Las Vegas was stressful for me, trying to plan for any eventuality that could occur to my family while I was out of town. The house was a mess, the kids were fussy and begging me not to leave, and our nanny was late. It was a chaotic morning. I raced to the airport and barely made it to the airport in time to catch my plane. I broke every speed limit law and dropped off my car with the airport valet. I ran through the airport and arrived at the gate just as they were closing the door to the jetway. I arrived in a puddle of sweat.

I made it on the plane and was ecstatic to find an aisle seat - 25C - still available. I sat down and began to settle in, planning to take advantage of the three-hour flight and catch up on some much-needed shut-eye. I started to fade as we took off and fell into a peaceful sleep. I was woken up a while later by the flight attendants and drink carts. I drank my sparkling water and ate the peanuts before shutting my eyes again. The pilot came on the PA system, encouraging us to check out the sights below us, as well as telling us we were about halfway to our destination.

A short while later, and before I could fall back asleep, the head flight attendant came on the PA system and asked in an urgent tone, "Is there a doctor on the plane?" I didn't immediately respond and looked around me in the cabin. No one stood up or raised their hand, including me. I sat frozen in my seat, trying to decide if I should respond to the plea for medical assistance.

I turned around and looked to see a man sitting in the seat behind me and across the aisle in 26D, being attended to by a flight attendant. He was of obvious Arab descent, and he looked very uncomfortable and sweaty. His once brown skin now looked decidedly pale and gray. I knew I had found the in-flight emergency, and he was sitting one row away. *Oh joy, what fun are we going to have today at 36,000 feet in the air?* I wondered, as I realized that I should probably volunteer my services.

"Asking again, is there a doctor on the plane? We have an emergency," a different flight attendant asked over the intercom with a bit more urgency in her voice. Given I was one row ahead of the flyer in question, I raised my hand with trepidation. I had little experience at that point with actively dying patients outside of a hospital, and zero experience with medical interventions six miles up in the air. Before I stood up from my seat, I prayed I wouldn't regret this decision to help this man.

After identifying myself as a doctor, I was immediately surrounded by three flight attendants, all looking to me for advice and direction. The passenger in question was now moaning and writhing in his seat, sweating profusely. I turned around in the aisle and introduced myself to the flight team, and also to the patient. A flight attendant introduced him to me as Mohammad and told me he was 56 years old.

"Hi, sir, my name is Dr. Casper. I am going to try and help you," I said.

Mid-flight emergencies are relatively rare, thankfully. The most common problems at elevation include neurologic events, such as seizures and strokes, which make up 41% of in-flight emergencies; followed by cardiac events at 27%. The change in the cabin air pressure and oxygen saturation can bring on these symptoms, and alcohol almost always makes these situations worse. Rarely, someone will die mid-flight.

"Help me!" Mohammad implored me as I stood in the aisle next to his seat. "I can't breathe. I feel like someone is sitting on my chest!" As he finished his sentence, a flight attendant handed me a large, plastic-wrapped bag full of medical goodies: an oxygen saturation monitor, a small oxygen tank, and a few first aid medications. I was then handed a stethoscope, a blood pressure cuff, gloves, and a mask for me. An EKG or defibrillator was not available on a plane at that time.

"We need to get Mohammad to an area where we can lay him down," I stated. Miraculously, and on a full flight, the team managed to clear three contiguous seats for Mohammad to rest, and for me to administer any treatments I could. I was very happy we did not have to lie on the floor of the aisle or the galley.

"How long do we have left on this flight?" I asked the nearest flight attendant.

"The captain says we are over halfway to Las Vegas. He needs to know as soon as possible if you would like him to fly back to Seattle, continue to Las Vegas, or land somewhere else sooner," the steward asked me.

Good Lord, how am I supposed to know what to do without an EKG or other sophisticated equipment? I wondered. Mohammad certainly looked like he was having a heart attack. To decide what we should do, I had to weigh factors such as Mohammad's condition, the flight duration, and the airport and hospital capabilities once we picked an airport to land in.

It now occurred to me that I had signed up all by myself to voluntarily be in charge of this suffering man. I felt completely alone and inept at that moment. I hoped I hadn't made a critical error in helping him so early in my tenure as a full-fledged physician. I wondered what the potential repercussions could be. I was counting on good Samaritan laws to prevail if things took a turn for the worse.

Good Samaritan laws protect individuals from legal liability who assist others in distress. This is provided they act in good faith, without gross negligence, and within their scope of training. The laws aim to encourage bystanders to help during emergencies, like what was occurring on the plane with Mohammad. In the U.S., all 50 states have some kind of good Samaritan law.

Good Samaritan laws typically cover first aid, CPR, or other emergency interventions. Helpers, like I was on the plane, must act voluntarily and without expectation of compensation. Some states limit protection to trained individuals, such as EMTs and physicians. Some states can actually apply penalties to people for *failing* to help someone in an emergency.

Limitations of protection under good Samaritan laws may apply if the helper is reckless, intoxicated, or exceeds their expertise. At that point, I was unclear of how the good Samaritan laws would apply to an in-flight emergency. But I hoped for the best outcome for both Mohammad and me, and proceeded with helping him.

As he laid down on the three seats, Mohammad was moaning loudly and clenching his fist over his heart, a classic sign of a heart attack. I listened to Mohammad's heart and lungs, took his blood pressure and pulse, and put oxygen on him. I continuously wiped his face of the sweat dripping from every pore. A flight attendant brought me two aspirin, which I put in his mouth and advised him to chew. I also placed an inch of nitro paste on his chest after taking his blood pressure.

These interventions provided significant relief to Mohammad, and we both calmed down a bit. After letting him rest a little while, I reassessed him and determined that he was stabilizing. I wiped the sweat from his face and reassured him that he was going to be okay. I now needed to decide how to direct the plane.

"Sir, where is home for you?" I queried, hoping his answer would help me decide what to advise the captain.

"I live in Las Vegas," Mohammad replied between soft moans.

Decision made. We would continue the current flight itinerary and land in Nevada. I informed the team, who let the captain know the plan. Additionally, I asked the team to be sure that EMS and an ambulance would meet us *on* the plane when we landed in Vegas. At this point, I prayed again that I had made the right decision and that Mohammad would make it alive to his destination.

I spent the next 90 minutes attending to Mohammad, trying to stay somewhat clean of his bodily fluids. He vomited at one point, fortunately not on me, and peed his pants. He remained uncomfortable for the rest of the flight, but much improved from the aspirin and repeated nitro paste. He remained conscious, and every oxygenated breath that he took gave me confidence that he could survive what was most likely a myocardial infarction.

In-flight medical emergencies happen in approximately 1/200 flights, making them more common than most people realize. Women experience these events 54% of the time, and the average age of a person experiencing a medical emergency in the air is 43. At the time of writing this book, most airplanes now have AEDs and access to telemedicine professionals on the ground. But unfortunately, statistics show that crews who call in flight for medical assistance on terra firma only get responses from doctors or nurses 40-50% of the time.

If the patient's condition is severe in flight, the decision to divert to a different airport is made approximately 10% of the time. But flight duration and airport capabilities must be considered. There is little use to land at an airport if there is not an associated and appropriate hospital nearby to handle the emergency.

Before we landed, the captain let the passengers know that they would need to exit at the rear of the plane. This was so that EMS could enter from the front to attend to Mohammad unobstructed with their stretcher. After landing in Las Vegas, I sat with Mohammad as passenger after passenger passed us by as they walked to the back of the plane to disembark via the stairs.

One of the last passengers to leave the plane, a middle-aged man, stopped at our row and held out his hand for me to shake. Surprised, and still with a dirty glove on, I reached out to shake his hand. He smiled at me as we shook hands and said, "We are *really* lucky to have nurses like you in this world."

A nurse? Did he really just call me a nurse? I thought to myself as I rolled my eyes. *Sir, I'm a fucking doctor who just spent nearly a decade of training to earn that title! Did you not hear the flight attendant call for a doctor? They didn't call for a nurse!* I was not amused, but I was too tired to correct him at that moment, realizing there was no point. My nerves were shot, and my adrenaline was waning from the intensity of managing Mohammad's care alone for the past hour and a half. I couldn't wait to get to my Las Vegas hotel and take a much-needed shower.

After the last passenger had deplaned, the EMS crew boarded the plane. I gave a history of the happenings during the flight to the nearest person I could find. I then stepped back from Mohammad as they skillfully extracted him from the plane and put him on a stretcher. I walked with the EMS and Mohammad until we reached the inside of the terminal, where we parted ways. I squeezed Mohammad's hand and said goodbye to him, reassuring him that he was in good hands. He thanked me profusely for the care I provided to him on the plane.

As a thank you for helping to save Mohammad's life on the flight, I received a $25 gift certificate from the airline toward another flight.

Interlogue

Physician, Heal Thyself

What Happens When the Healer Needs Healing?

As I have mentioned previously in this book, physicians are expected to exhibit superhuman capabilities at times. Combined with long hours, little sleep, and an avalanche of medical information to learn and be competent at. But what happens when the healer needs healing?

When doctors get sick, their knowledge and access to healthcare networks can shape their experience. Doctors may self-diagnose or treat minor ailments themselves. They use their expertise to manage their symptoms or self-prescribe medications if legally permissible.

For example, a doctor with a cold might take over-the-counter remedies, knowing exactly which drug is needed to relieve their symptoms. However, for serious conditions, they usually seek care from colleagues. They seek care either informally (e.g., casually consulting with a trusted peer,) or formally, such as properly visiting a specialist as a patient.

Doctors face unique pressures. Due to demanding schedules and a sense of duty, they often work through mild illnesses, and sometimes major illnesses, potentially delaying their own care and treatment. A 2018 study in the *Journal of the American Medical Association* (*JAMA*) shows that physicians are less likely to take sick leave than other professionals, with 60% reporting working in patient care while ill themselves.

Working as a physician while sick stems from workplace culture (e.g., doctors themselves are not supposed to call in sick,) or fear of burdening already overworked colleagues. When doctors work while ill, several consequences can arise, impacting their own health, their patients' health, and the healthcare system in general.

Sick doctors can spread infectious diseases, especially respiratory illnesses like the flu or COVID-19. Physicians who work while sick increase the risk of transmission in high-contact environments like hospitals and outpatient clinics. This can endanger their colleagues and staff, as well as vulnerable patients, such as the immunocompromised or elderly.

Illness of any kind can impair a physician's cognitive and physical abilities. Fatigue, fever, or pain can reduce a doctor's focus, potentially leading to errors in diagnosis, treatment, or documentation. A 2019 *British Medical Journal* study noted that physicians working while unwell (known as presenteeism) correlates with a higher likelihood of medical mistakes, compromising patient safety.

Presenteeism refers to the situation where employees come to work, but they are not fully productive due to illness, stress, or personal issues. Essentially, the employee is physically present, but their performance is compromised. This leads to decreased productivity and potential negative impacts on the workplace. Presenteeism is the opposite of absenteeism, where employees are absent from work.

Working while sick delays recovery and can exacerbate conditions. For example, a doctor with a viral infection might develop complications like bacterial pneumonia if they don't rest and seek the appropriate treatment. Chronic presenteeism also contributes to burnout, with a 2021 *Mayo Clinic Proceedings* study linking presenteeism to higher rates of stress and mental health issues among physicians.

Healthcare culture often discourages physicians from taking sick leave - or even maternity leave - due to staffing shortages or fear of seeming unreliable to their coworkers. This is true throughout medical school, as I experienced, residency, and full-fledged practice. It is especially seen in high-pressure settings like emergency medicine and surgical specialties. A 2020 *Academic Medicine* survey found 70% of doctors felt pressure to work despite illness, perpetuating the cycle of presenteeism.

Doctors are not explicitly expected to never get sick, as illness is a natural part of being human. However, workplace culture, systemic pressures, and their role as healthcare providers create an implicit expectation for doctors to minimize sick days or work through an illness.

Doctors are often seen as pillars of resilience, with a professional culture that prioritizes patient care over their personal health. A majority of physicians work while sick, driven by a sense of duty to their patients or fear of letting down colleagues and health systems. This culture discourages taking sick leave, especially in understaffed settings where physician absences can significantly disrupt patient care. In my experience, patients rarely understand when their own doctor's appointments are cancelled due to the physician's illness.

While policies differ around the U.S., many healthcare systems expect doctors to avoid spreading illness. Some hospitals and clinics have sick leave protocols, requiring physicians to stay home if they are contagious (e.g., with a fever or respiratory symptoms). But enforcement is inconsistent, and many physicians still work while ill.

Mental health conditions, such as depression and anxiety, also play a significant role. A 2021 *Mayo Clinic Proceedings* study estimated that 20-30% of doctors experience clinically significant depression at some point in their career, and women are at higher risk. This is significantly higher than the general population risk of depression of 17-20%. But most often, physicians are hesitant to seek help due to the stigma of seeking mental healthcare or licensing concerns. The risk of major depression can be exacerbated by the high-stress environments, long shifts, and little rest, all of which are prevalent in medicine.

Major depression, anxiety disorders, and substance use disorders (particularly alcohol and pills) are frequently reported. Doctors face pressure to appear infallible, with stigmas around seeking mental healthcare. Mental health conditions, particularly depression and anxiety, are among the leading causes of disability claims for physicians. This can lead to extended leaves away from their jobs, or even a career change altogether.

Physician burnout is a significant risk and affects 40-60% of physicians, depending on the specialty. Burnout is characterized by emotional exhaustion, depersonalization, and a reduced sense of accomplishment. While burnout itself is not classified as a clinical diagnosis in the DSM-5, it is a major issue for physicians. It often precedes a diagnosis of depression or a disability claim. A 2019 *BMJ* study found doctors with burnout were twice as likely to make errors in their work.

Physician burnout stems from a variety of factors. Long hours - often 60-80 hours/week - can add up over time and contribute to exhaustion and burnout. Likewise, high patient loads, administrative burdens, and life-or-death decision-making in the job all contribute to the problem. Emergency medicine, surgery, and critical care physicians report higher burnout rates due to intense workloads. More humane specialties, like dermatology and pathology, often report lower burnout rates.

Another revealing statistic regards a physician's paid time off (PTO). A 2025 study in *JAMA Network Open* revealed that 70% of primary care physicians work while on vacation. This only makes their risk of burnout, anxiety, and depression even worse. Overall, a study in 2025 by *MedCentral* showed that 35% of all physicians are considering leaving the practice of medicine due to burnout, the number one reason.

Burnout and depression correlate with medical errors, reduced patient satisfaction, and costly higher turnover of staff. Mental health issues can lead to substance abuse, relationship strain, or suicide. According to a 2020 *American Journal of Psychiatry* report, suicide rates are higher among doctors than in other professions. Male physicians have a

1.4 times higher risk of suicide, and female physicians have up to 2.3 times higher risk of suicide than the general population.

A 2021 study estimated that one of every 15 doctors has considered suicide at some point in their career. This is a significant occupational hazard when compared to the lifetime risk of suicide in the general population of 1/200 people. In 2024, with over 1.1 million practicing physicians in the U.S., this amounts to approximately 75,000 physicians who have contemplated ending their lives at some point in their career. This is a staggering number, and a statistic that is rarely discussed in medicine. The risk of a physician committing suicide is truly a very real occupational hazard.

The number of physicians in private practice has steadily declined every year as corporations continue to acquire solo practices in all specialties. This has significantly changed the landscape of employment for physicians. In 2012, 60% of physicians were in private practice (where they have control of their own schedule).

But by 2024, only 42% of physicians were self-employed, signifying a significant trend toward corporate medicine employment and less autonomy for the physician. Not being in total control of their schedule contributes substantially to physician stress and burnout.

Workplace violence is a real and severe threat to those in the medical profession. Healthcare workers make up only 10% of the workforce in the U.S., but they experience 48% of non-fatal injuries while at work. This has led to a significant presence of armed law enforcement officers in healthcare settings. According to a recent study in Stateline.org, at least 29 states now allow hospitals to have their own police force. This ever-present risk of violence while at work significantly adds to the stress that physicians feel.

Another contributor to stress and financial overwhelm is the crushing debt that physicians take on for payment of medical school. The average debt in 2024 across all medical school graduates in the U.S. was $212,000. This debt, which can haunt physicians for decades after completion of medical school, is a significant contributor to the stress that physicians feel.

Additionally, significant pay gaps are found between physician specialties that contribute to the demoralization of physicians. For example, in 2024, surgical specialists earned 87% *more* money than primary care physicians. This is an astonishing figure when you consider the fact that the workload and hours of these two specialties are quite similar.

A recent study revealed that 85% of physicians feel they are overworked, and a staggering 66% of all physicians are considering a job change or early retirement. As I have shared throughout this book, the challenges facing physicians are many - whether in medical school, residency, or post-graduate practice. Oftentimes, the barriers to getting care for oneself, whether real or perceived, are a significant deterrent due to a multitude of factors.

So, what is a physician to do when *they* get sick, *really sick?* What if the healer needs healing themselves? What follows is the story of my own diagnosis of and treatment for cancer.

Chapter 29
The Dreaded "C" Word

In 2017, I retired from the practice of medicine. I was completely burnt out and ready to leave the day-to-day stress of being a physician. I had already established two other companies outside of medicine, and I decided to shift my life focus to these two business endeavors.

One morning in 2019, while in Malibu, California, I had a melanic stool, seemingly out of nowhere. I had had a "clean" colonoscopy just 18 months before, so this was completely unexpected. As a former physician, I instinctively knew this bloody stool was not good at all - but I lacked the energy or desire to pursue it further. I figured, incorrectly and due to my denial of the facts in the toilet bowl, that it was an isolated incident that I could ignore.

Mind you, if one of my patients had ever reported having a bloody stool to me when I was in practice, I would have made sure that they saw a gastroenterologist as soon as possible. But, with my focus elsewhere, I chose to ignore what I saw. I flushed the evidence, and any concerns, down the toilet and carried on with my life.

A few weeks later, and back at home in Seattle after I visited Malibu, I had the same problem, only much worse. The blood was so dark and filled the toilet bowl. Given that I was more alert and focused at that time, I understood the medical gravity of what I was seeing in the toilet bowl. Due to my relatively recent clean colonoscopy, I assumed the bleed must have been from a stomach ulcer or some other benign colon condition. Colon cancer was the last thing on my mind, and no one in my family had ever had cancer of any type.

I immediately called my gastroenterologist's office, where I had had the colonoscopy, and they scheduled me for a same-day appointment. I met with a physician whom I had never met before and showed him the picture I had taken of the blood in the toilet.

"Liz, thank you for bringing in this picture. As they say, a picture is worth a thousand words, and in your case, it is," Dr. Chow said with a very serious look on his face. "You have colon cancer, until proven otherwise," he said bluntly and without softening the blow.

"Colon cancer?" I replied, shocked to hear the words come out of his mouth. "Are you kidding me? I had a clean colonoscopy with this office less than two years ago!"

"Yes, I know," he paused. "Honestly, Liz, we must have missed the cancer when we performed the colonoscopy," he confessed.

Missed the freaking cancer? You're not serious! I thought to myself. *How can this be happening to me? It just can't be cancer!*

"I am going to admit you to the hospital tonight. It looks like you are losing a large amount of blood, and that can be very dangerous, as you know," he continued. "I will get you tucked in for the night, and then one of my colleagues will scope you after you complete a colon prep. You will need an endoscopy of your stomach and a colonoscopy of your colon. Please head to the hospital now, and I will see you there in a couple of hours," he finished.

My head was reeling from what Dr. Chow had just told me. I walked to my car in a daze and drove the too-short distance to the hospital. Once there, I checked in. The admission process did not go smoothly after I informed the intake secretary that I would not accept any blood products. They assumed that I was a Jehovah's Witness (I am not) and hassled me mercilessly about my decision. I was even threatened with potential denial of my workup and surgery if I did not agree to accept blood. But I knew my rights, and I stuck to my guns: no blood for me.

The receptionist finally relented and checked me into the hospital. Afterward, she informed me that she was going to order an ethics consult for me so that "we" could discuss the blood issue further. Soon thereafter, an orderly came with a wheelchair and whisked me away to room #303. They ordered a STAT hemoglobin and hematocrit, which showed that I had indeed lost a lot of blood. But, given my young age and overall good health, my numbers were not low enough to warrant the blood transfusion discussion again.

My decision to decline blood was written boldly on the dry-erase board in my hospital room, causing every nurse and doctor who saw me to inquire why. I found myself repeating over and over, "Because I choose to decline. No, it's not for religious reasons, it's just my preference." *Why did everyone seem to want to give me someone else's blood?* I wondered. As they tucked me into bed for the night, my blood pressure dropped to 80/40. After several litres of normal saline brought my pressure up, my hematocrit fell two more points. Steadfast, I continued to decline blood products.

I had to wait for two days in the hospital to complete the "colonoscopy prep" before the scopes could be performed. If you haven't had the pleasure of going through this pre-op procedure, you really are missing out on a good time. It involves drinking a disgusting fluid that will eventually clear out your entire system, bowel movement by bowel movement. You drink the drink and continue to defecate until your poop is nothing but clear liquid. Then, and only then, are you ready for the scoping of your stomach and intestines, or surgery on your colon.

On my fourth hospital day, I met with another gastroenterologist who would be performing the scopes in the OR under general anesthesia. He rattled off the consent for the procedures like he was in a great hurry, and I signed the paperwork literally as I was being wheeled into the endoscopy suite. The next memory I had was waking up in the recovery room with the same doctor attempting to show me the pictures he took during the procedures of my insides.

"See here, Liz," he started as he flipped through the pages of thumbnail pictures, stopping to show me one in particular. "See this mass? It's about four centimeters in diameter and is partially obstructing your lower colon," he finished.

As I came out of the anaesthesia, I took the papers from him to get a closer look at the mass. "That's not cancer, that looks like a fungus!" I exclaimed.

"A fungus?" he asked in disbelief. "It's definitely not a fungus, Liz. It's cancer," he finished.

"I guess we will have to agree to disagree. Now what?" I asked in my near delirious state.

"Now, we will get you scheduled for surgery. I've already called the best gastrointestinal general surgeon in our hospital. Dr. Colon will come by and see you later today." With that, I was wheeled on a stretcher back to my room.

I met the surgeon later that day and found him to be an unusually delightful older man with a great bedside manner, out of keeping for most surgeons. He explained the surgery he had planned in great detail and spoke to me as though I were still his physician colleague. He let me know that, in addition to removing the mass, he would be searching for adjacent lymph nodes in the mesentery and sending them to pathology for evaluation and further staging of my cancer.

I signed the consent for surgery, and he let me know I was on the schedule for the first thing the next morning. At that moment, the hardest thing was remaining NPO (no food or drink) for what was now five days in the hospital. I was *so* hungry. I had lost so much weight during my pre-diagnosis, hypermetabolic state, that I began to look a bit anorexic myself. Bones protruded beneath my skin, and my face looked drawn and gaunt. I couldn't wait to start eating again after surgery, even if it was hospital food.

The next morning, a nurse woke me up at six a.m. with a valium. After taking a quick shower to wash my hair and body, an orderly came to my room with a stretcher to take me to surgery. Once in the pre-op area, Dr. Colon and the anaesthesiologist greeted me and explained the procedure once again. I let them know I was allergic to certain drugs and requested propofol and fentanyl, which they unanimously agreed to give me. They wheeled me into the OR, and the ballet began, only this time it was *me* on the table.

"Okay, Liz," the anaesthesiologist said to me as he put an oxygen mask on me and began to inject the propofol into my IV. "Please count backward from ten," he instructed as he continued the infusion into my arm.

"Ten, nine, eight, sev….," That's as far as I got before the amazing drug washed over me like warm sunlight on a cold day. My body felt relaxed and euphoric as I fell asleep peacefully. I woke up hours later in the post-op recovery area without any nausea due to my choice of anaesthetic drugs. As soon as I was fully awake, a nurse handed me ice chips to munch on as I waited for the surgeon to come speak with me.

"Well, Liz, we found and removed the entire cancer from your colon. It looks like you might have some cancer in the adjacent lymph nodes, so we removed them too and have sent them to pathology for staging. I will come see you tonight in your room before I leave for the day," Dr. Colon finished.

"Thank you so much, Dr. Colon," I replied before I fell back asleep.

I spent several more days in the hospital recovering from the extensive surgery and getting stronger. My family and friends brought me delicious food and treats, which I gratefully ate, and beautiful flowers to brighten my room. Every day, I felt stronger and healthier. Finally, on day 11, I was able to be discharged home.

Chapter 30
Cancer, Chemo, & COVID

After my surgery, I had to wait a couple of weeks for the pathology report to come back. I was given a stage of 3b colon cancer, as one of my adjacent mesenteric lymph nodes was positive. My surgeon recommended that I visit with an oncologist, and gave me the name of a couple of people he knew and respected. A retired physician friend of mine, who had overcome two different cancer diagnoses in her life, recommended one oncologist in particular on the list. After researching him a bit online, I placed a call to his office to make an appointment.

As a medical student, I didn't learn too much about chemotherapy. As a resident, I had never rotated through an oncology office, so I had little to prepare me for my first visit to the oncologist.

Simultaneous to my first visit to the oncologist, the U.S. had begun and exceeded the "Two Weeks to Flatten the

Curve" COVID-19 lockdowns. This meant that I would have to go to my chemo appointment all alone, as visitors were no longer welcome due to the perceived increased risk of infection. Given that chemotherapy patients are already significantly immunosuppressed, the infection control in their office was as tight as Fort Knox.

I looked up the address on Google Maps and drove myself to my first visit. The building was massive, and the parking lot was huge and full of cars. I approached the front doors and was greeted by an assistant handing out masks, gloves, and antibacterial disinfectant. *Quite an entrance,* I thought to myself. Once inside the huge building, I stood in line, six feet apart from the next unlucky patient, and waited to be called to the extensive reception desk. There were six employees slowly checking in a long line of patients. *Note to self: arrive earlier next time!*

The vast waiting area was packed with patients of all ages, who honestly looked like they were waiting to die. Wheelchairs and walkers were the norm, as were hats, wigs, and fabric covering heads with chemotherapy-induced hair loss. Everyone around me looked sick, really sick, and the general color of everyone's skin was some shade of gray. I didn't see one healthy-looking person in the entire area, and wondered if I would end up looking like them in the not-too-distant future. *I sure hope not!* I said to myself as I began to feel depressed and question my decision to get chemotherapy.

I finally was able to check in and was then told to take a seat and wait to be called. I waited for about 15 minutes before my name was called. "Liz Casper!" a young woman yelled into the overflowing waiting room. *Did she really just call me by my first and last name? Breaking HIPAA rules?* I was horrified and shocked that they would do that.

I got up from my seat and followed the girl through a door to another part of the building. As I did so, I politely reminded her to only use my first name in the future. She seemed clueless and unconcerned, so I decided I would speak to the physician himself about the breach in privacy.

We walked around the massive building until we reached the area where my physician, Dr. Chemo, had his office and exam rooms. I was weighed in the hallway on a very public scale with people all around me. I was then placed in a sterile exam room. There, I waited for another 20 minutes before Dr. Chemo breezed into the room.

"Hi Liz, I'm Dr. Chemo," he said as he reached his gloved hand to shake my own. "Nice to meet you. I'm sorry it's under these circumstances."

"Hi, Dr. Chemo, nice to meet you," I replied. "I'm a retired physician, so you can 'talk shop' to me. You've also successfully treated a physician friend of mine, Dr. Gardner. She highly recommended you."

"That's great. Dr. Gardner is a wonderful colleague of mine. I understand you are here today to discuss chemotherapy?" he asked.

"Yes, I recently had colon cancer removed, and my surgeon recommended that I speak with you and get your opinion on the matter," I replied. "If you don't mind, I'd like to include my parents in this conversation. I brought two phones and I'd like to FaceTime them while we talk." At that time, you could only FaceTime one person at a time, so I needed two phones to include both of my parents.

"That's not a problem at all. It's actually a really great idea, Liz," he stated. "I will suggest it to my other patients as we navigate this pandemic situation."

I called both of my parents on the video app, and we began our visit. "Hi, Mom. Hi, Dad," Dr. Chemo said after all the electronic connections had been made to my parents. "We are here today to discuss whether or not Liz should start chemotherapy. I am happy to hear your input, but the decision is ultimately hers."

Dr. Chemo then went on to describe both my cancer, its stage, and the recommended chemotherapy for it. I, myself, was very hesitant to commence chemo as I had heard horror stories about it from my patients and friends over the years. And Dr. Colon had indicated he had successfully removed all of the cancer in my body. As such, I challenged Dr. Chemo to give me a specific reason *why* I should go through with the now-described brutal, six-month regimen.

"Well, Liz, with your type and stage of cancer, without chemo, you have a 30% five-year survival rate. With this chemotherapy, that statistic changes to a 70% five-year survival rate." I thought long and hard about those statistics and solicited opinions from my parents. Ultimately, I decided to commence a six-month regimen of chemo. I would have infusions of the recommended drugs every three weeks for a total of eight infusions.

Dr. Chemo then went on to describe the side effects I could expect to see: hair loss, nausea, and weight loss were essentially a given. He went on to describe the real risk of very painful changes of sensation in my hands and feet, which may be permanent. He told me that I should avoid situations where my hands and feet could get cold, as that change in temperature of my extremities would make the pain much worse. I tried to imagine what it would be like and wondered what really awaited me.

Before I left the visit with Dr. Chemo, I asked him what kind of a diet I should follow, assuming there would be research on diet and colon cancer. He looked at me quizzically and indicated that there were no dietary restrictions or changes that he could recommend to increase my chances of a cure. He implied that my colon cancer was unrelated to diet, and diet was unrelated to my chemotherapy regimen. I was surprised at his answer and decided I would do my own research once I got home. True to his word, there really weren't any definitive recommendations from any good studies that I could find. Going on my "gut instinct", pun intended, I did my best to eat a high-fiber, low sugar, organic diet.

My every three-week infusions of chemotherapy would take about a week to fully take effect in my body. I was told that in these three-week intervals, I could expect to feel my best during the third week and just before a new infusion, when the chemo was nearly washed out of my system. *Wow, two weeks that are going to suck, and maybe one good week, to be repeated eight times over the next 24 weeks? This sounds horrible! Have I made the right decision?* I wondered. At that moment, COVID-19 and the lockdowns seemed to be a bit of a blessing, as I could recuperate at home and wouldn't have to worry about going to my office. I would also have less exposure to a contagious illness while in my chemo-induced, immunosuppressed state.

Dr. Chemo then let me know that he needed to have my blood drawn to look at a tumor marker called CEA, or carcinoembryonic antigen. CEA is a protein marker used in cancer diagnosis and monitoring, particularly for colon cancer. We would get a baseline figure, then monitor the CEA at each visit with him. He also said I would need to get a baseline CT scan with contrast of my abdomen. I would get this CT scan repeated every three months for two years; then every six months for an additional three years. After five years of monitoring my bloodwork and CT scans, I would be considered "cured" from my cancer.

A CT scan employs a lot of radiation and can only pick up cancerous lesions that are one centimeter or greater in size. As a former physician, I wondered *why* they only employed a CT scan for monitoring, versus an MRI, which has no radiation exposure. It seemed odd and intuitively incorrect to me. I couldn't see how continually exposing an immunocompromised cancer patient to so much radiation was a good thing, but Dr. Chemo was resolute about the protocol.

Finally, Dr. Chemo recommended that I go back to Dr. Colon and have a port placed in my chest to enable easy access for chemotherapy. We hung up the FaceTime calls with my parents, and Dr. Chemo completed a thorough physical exam on me. As he helped me up from the exam table, he said, "Follow me, I'll take you to our scheduling department."

We left the exam room together and walked to the opposite side of the massive building, where there was a back-office scheduling department, cloaked in privacy. This was in contrast to the very public reception area that had greeted me. Before leaving the building, I made an appointment to begin my chemotherapy program, about one month hence, and after most of the healing of my colon and port was complete.

I weaved my way back through the massive building and passed a packed waiting room before exiting to the parking lot. There was a long line of patients extending out the front door. I was impressed, but not in a good way, by all of the people seeking care for cancer. It was the busiest clinic I had ever witnessed in my nearly 25 years in medicine.

As I left the building, I removed my mask and gloves and threw them into a garbage can before getting in my car and driving home. I hoped I had made the right decision regarding chemotherapy, but I really wasn't sure at that point. Once home, I called Dr. Colon and arranged to have a port placed as soon as possible.

Chapter 31
Commencing Chemo

As most people know, the two weeks to flatten the COVID curve turned into a years-long lockdown and complete disruption of our lives. My businesses in Seattle had all been temporarily closed, so I was stuck at home, all alone, to recover from the chemotherapy. I guess in hindsight, it was a bit of a blessing. As the chemotherapy was destroying my immune system, I was exposed to fewer illnesses. I spent my time at home working on creative projects and busying myself. I tried to keep my mind off the brutal journey that awaited me in the chemotherapy room at Dr. Chemo's office.

The day of my first chemo treatment arrived far too quickly. I had decided that I was going to wear a beautiful red outfit on each visit. "Fighting red," I told myself. I was going to tackle this stupid cancer and chemo, and *win*. I promised myself that I would wear this bright red outfit at each of my eight visits, as a statement that *I* was winning, not the cancer.

I drove to the center, and I found a parking place in the packed lot and waited in line to be checked in again. At the door, I was again given a mask and gloves. This time, when I checked into the clinic, the receptionist directed me to go upstairs to the second floor of the massive building. Once there, I checked in with another receptionist who instructed me to wait in an adjacent, smaller waiting room. This was the chemotherapy waiting area, I soon learned.

I took my seat in the room and waited for what seemed like a long time. Several people, who looked like they were at death's door, were called back into the chemo room before me. I was terrified at what I was witnessing: no one smiled, and all looked exhausted and depressed. They all looked so sick that they may not make it through the treatment. I texted my mom and told her I wanted to change my mind. I did not want to end up looking or feeling like these people appeared. They truly looked like they were one step away from their grave. *How is this living?* I asked myself.

My mom encouraged me to continue with the plan for chemotherapy and tried to calm me down, as though she were there with me. After about another 15 minutes, my name was finally called. "Liz Casper!" a nurse said loudly as she held open the chemo door. *Unfuckingbelievable! Why are they using my full name? Does HIPAA not exist in Oncology?* I wondered again.

As I walked with the nurse through the door, I reiterated, "Please do not use my full name!"

The nurse laughed off my concerns as though what I had said didn't matter, and led me through an enormous, light-filled room. The chemo room was completely packed with wall-to-wall people, in what looked like various stages of dying. It kind of looked like a fluorescent-lit gymnasium with office cubicles, but instead of desks, there were IV poles and reclining chairs. They were stacked so closely together that there was literally no way to have a treatment in private.

I could hear every conversation around me between the nurses and patients. I was shocked by how the patients were thrown together, and conversations with staff and patients were initiated within earshot of multiple other people. Again, I felt like my privacy really didn't matter to them, just the treatment protocol. I started my first infusion in a very bad mood.

Once I was settled in a recliner, a very kind and energetic nurse came to greet me. She accessed the port in my chest and explained the procedure and what I could expect afterwards. The infusion would take approximately four hours, and I might begin to feel symptoms before it was completed. The room had a makeshift kitchen in it, with coffee and snacks available. But because I was tied to an immovable IV pole, I wasn't able to partake, and no assistance with nutrition from the kitchen was offered. I made a mental note to grab sustenance before my next infusion.

The four-hour chemo treatment dragged on and on, and I didn't appreciate being packed in like a sardine with other patients receiving treatment. Once the medicine had been completely emptied from the IV bag and into my system, it took another 30 minutes before any nurse had the time to assist me and let me go home. They were so busy that it looked like an emergency room on steroids. I couldn't wait to leave.

After my first treatment, I went home and waited for the side effects to start. On day three, I started to feel like I had the flu, with general malaise, nausea, and vomiting. By day five, I could no longer feel my fingertips or toes. And with exposure to any cold (air or water), I experienced extremely painful shocks and a burning sensation in my extremities. The pain was excruciating, and I prayed it would not become a permanent fixture in my life.

Weeks one and two after the chemo were the worst, and true to Dr. Chemo's words, week three was the best, but still horrible. Usually, the day before my next treatment was when I felt my best, and it was hard to continue treatment, given how painful and life-altering the side effects were. It's hard for me to describe how horrible chemotherapy makes you feel. I literally felt like the walking dead at times.

I somehow made it through the eight sessions of chemo, as I continued to have significant pain and neuropathy 24/7 in my hands and feet. At my bi-monthly visits with Dr. Chemo, we monitored my decreasing CEA, and I was also monitored with the CT scans, which remained clear.

I ended up losing about half of my hair, and most of it turned snow white and curly when it grew back. Wigs became a familiar friend as I left the house more frequently, as some of the COVID-19 restrictions started to lift. I lost quite a bit more weight as I was going through the chemo, but I tried to eat only healthy, organic food. I researched colon cancer almost obsessively, and I took a daily concoction of supplements that were reported to help. I was resolute that I would be cured at the end of this whole ordeal.

Today, six years from my diagnosis, I remain cancer-free and healthy. I have decided that if cancer should ever find my body again, I would most likely not go through chemotherapy. It was, by far, the worst thing I have ever experienced in medicine as a patient.

Chapter 32
Near-Death Experience

In the months after my diagnosis and treatment for colon cancer, I was extremely ill from the chemotherapy, as you might imagine. At times, my days and nights were indistinguishable. The hallucinations and delusions, from the cancer and the side effects from the chemotherapy, were vivid, realistic, and a constant companion. When they eased their grip on me, I was able to function somewhat normally for a short period of time.

Being a former physician, I had become quite familiar with death and dying when it happened to my patients. I was even given the name "Dr. Death" by my hospital comrades because I was so comfortable with death and dying. So comfortable that I often would sit with my patients as they transitioned to a better place. Personally, however, I had had very little experience with death, other than the usual loss of grandparents. And I had never really considered my own death, and what that might look/feel/be like. All that changed one day as I became extremely sick from my sixth chemotherapy session.

Before my diagnosis of colon cancer, I had just moved into a newly built house and was having trouble adjusting to my new surroundings, given the state I was in at that time. In the recent weeks since the move, I had difficulty staying grounded, often popping in and out of an awake or delirious state. All I knew was that I was getting more ill by the day and was losing touch with reality.

One evening, after a particularly difficult treatment day filled with frightening visions of death, I truly didn't know how I could go on. The chemotherapy made me feel so sick that I felt my life was coming to an end. I wasn't sure I would make it through the night. After vomiting up what little dinner I had eaten, I decided to go to bed and see if I could wake up to a better situation. I laid down on the bed and waited for sleep to arrive. I shut my eyes and was quickly taken on a journey that changed my life forever.

I was transported through the proverbial black tunnel, heading in a counter-clockwise circular spiral towards a yellow light in the distance, awaiting me at the end of the tunnel. The journey to the light was marked by a beautiful aroma and weightless feeling, almost as if I were flying. It felt like I was dancing through the tunnel, and I could feel the "gravity" pulling me through and towards the bright, yellow light. In hindsight, it felt like how a black hole or wormhole might be described.

At the end of the tunnel, I exited, now without any identifiable human characteristics. I entered a vast area in the sky where I met with a golden being at a location that looked like the "pearly gates." Once there, I was greeted by the being - an amorphous spirit, really - who welcomed me into my new life. The being let me know that they were there to conduct my life review, as it was required to be allowed through the gates that I saw before me.

The being took their time as they looked over my life that seemed to be written on some sort of an amorphous scroll. They analyzed my life silently and thoroughly. Finally, the being looked up at me and said telepathically, "You've been through so much in your lifetime on earth. But you have been *good. Really good.*"

I wasn't sure what I should say to that positive assessment, but I was grateful that it was good. In reply, again with non-verbal communication, I said, "I know!" when what I really wanted to say was "no shit, Sherlock." Somehow, swearing at the gates of what looked like Heaven didn't seem appropriate. It felt really good to have my earthly modus operandi validated by this amorphous spirit.

The being gave me a big smile as they put an energetic arm around my shoulders. They gently led me toward and through what looked like white marble gates. I began to move forward with the being as we floated effortlessly through the air. But before I knew where we were going, the being vanished into thin air, leaving me all alone in a new area.

In front of me, there was a scene like no other I have ever witnessed before on earth. The colors were vivid and unlike anything I had ever experienced. Gardens upon gardens lay out before me with the most beautiful plants, trees, flowers and fauna that I had ever seen. Animals, like dogs, cats, cows, deer, and birds, were everywhere and interacting peacefully with each other. There were beautiful waterfalls, and crystal-clear ponds and lakes everywhere I looked.

The light all around me was the brightest and most beautiful light I had ever seen, but it did not hurt my eyes. It was like looking into the sun without any difficulty or harm. It was pure illumination, and it was clear that no darkness could reside there. I was inundated with the pure, yellow-white light. The only emotion I could feel at that point was that of overwhelming Love. Pure Love.

I looked around the gardens and became aware of other energies that were near me. They weren't human, but they were definitely living beings, and occasionally their energies would morph in and out of human-like characteristics, such as hands and faces. While I didn't see anyone or anything that I could identify for certain, there was an odd familiarity with some of the beings, and I was comforted simply by being near them.

A short time later - I'm really not sure how long because time didn't exist there - I was enveloped by a being with a very masculine energy. He took me into his arms energetically and welcomed me to Heaven.

"Welcome, Liz. Congratulations, you made it through the game! We are so glad you are here," the being said, again telepathically. It blended our two energies and began to slowly sway with me to a beautiful, symphonic melody. I felt an incredible sense of peace, joy, and happiness wash over me as we continued our psychic dance. The being held me gently, and at times it seemed that our two energies became one. I was overcome with joy by the gentle interaction, and the only way that I can describe this event is pure bliss. I didn't want our psychic dance to end. Ever.

As we continued to slowly move in unison, the being pulled away from me and looked deeply into my soul and asked me, not with words, but by his wordless energy, "Where do you want to go next?"

I looked at him quizzically and telepathically replied, "What do you mean?"

"Where do you want to go? You can go anywhere you want. You have graduated from that game on earth," he replied. Meaning, I could choose to go anywhere in the universe and begin a new game.

"I want to go back to earth!" I replied reflexively and without forethought.

"Earth?" he asked in a *very* surprised tone.

"Yes, earth," I continued as he pulled me back closer to him.

"*Why* would you *want* to go back to earth?" he said telepathically, and in disbelief and shock.

"*Why*? Because I'm not done yet!" I replied.

As soon as I finished my telepathic reply, I was immediately ripped away from the being's embrace and transported back to earth. I returned in a clockwise fashion back through the dark tunnel from which I had arrived in heaven. When I next opened my eyes, on earth, I quickly checked the clock. I noticed that no time had passed while I went on my psychic, ethereal journey.

Although it's been a few years since this experience, it changed me forever. I do not fear death in the slightest. To be frank, it is quite alluring at times, given what life here on earth can throw at you. This otherworld experience certainly gave me a great deal of comfort as I faced my potential death sentence with the diagnosis of colon cancer. I truly believe it helped me remain peaceful and serene as I went through and completed the brutal regimen of chemotherapy.

So, the former "Dr. Death" herself had had a near-death experience. As Jim Morrison sang, "Break on through, to the other side," I did, and it was good. *Really good.* Now, I can truly say, "*Life,* here on earth, is Good." Because I've seen the other side, and it is something to look forward to.

Chapter 33
A Brighter Future

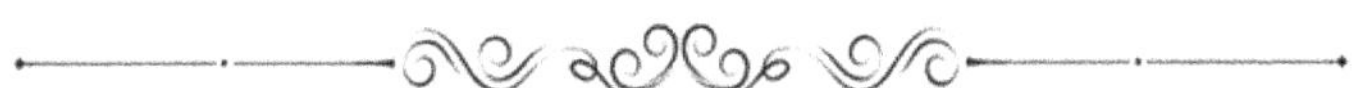

Becoming a physician is one of the hardest professional pursuits one can achieve. Academic rigor, exceptional effort, and unwavering commitment to the profession are required. Preparing for entry to medical school can be a decade-long pursuit, often beginning in high school or earlier. The dream of medical school and residency can take another decade or more to complete. Generally, only the most dedicated and resilient make it through and ultimately can put M.D. behind their name.

Shockingly, over the past several decades, there has been a systematic dismantling of our education system in the U.S. Requirements to meet academic milestones and standards have gone away, and have been replaced by equity of grades for all, regardless of effort or interest. Competition has become a four-letter word. And somehow we must now all agree that we are all equal winners in the game of life, despite often unequal effort and/or intellect. By graduating children and young adults from schools and institutions of higher learning, without qualifications to back up the purported achievements, we weaken society as a whole and put our collective future in peril.

Medical school admissions in the U.S. continue to demand strong academic credentials, but they are changing the way that they evaluate applicants. They are focusing on diversity and a more holistic approach to admissions. Medical schools are assessing competency via means other than grades and academic achievements. GPAs of medical school applicants before admission to medical school average 3.86. And the median Medical College Admission Test (MCAT) score is 512, denoting proficiency in the basic sciences and math.

Acceptance rates of applications to medical school have declined from a difficult 10.5% to a current and dismal 6.6%. At the time of writing this book, approximately 40 medical schools had deemphasized the MCATs. Instead, choosing to focus on other qualities such as clinical experience, community service, and personal attributes. This is being done to better align with the need for compassionate and diverse physicians to serve an increasingly diverse population.

The average student, even with all the requirements met, usually applies to 15-25 medical schools to gain admission. This is an expensive and time-consuming endeavor. And many people have to apply over and over, year after year, to be admitted to a medical school, somewhere, *anywhere*. The total number of medical school applicants has been steadily *decreasing* year-over-year, with approximately 60,000 applicants in 2024 to 155 schools.

This decline in medical school applications is multifactorial, with financial burdens at the top of the list. The average graduate from medical school amasses $200,000 or more in debt at the end of their four-year education. Additionally, fewer prospective students are attracted to a profession that requires extensive and expensive training, long hours, and challenging work conditions. This is especially true as physician compensation has not kept pace with the cost and total debt from medical school that continues to rise year after year.

Eliminating, or even lowering, general academic standards in our society has far-reaching implications and devastating consequences. This impacts the workforce and society in general. Removing standards affects foundational skills in math, reading, and science, which are required to succeed in medical school and as a physician. This produces "graduates" who are unprepared for complex problem-solving and even employment.

Some graduating students today cannot read cursive, cannot tell time on a non-digital clock, and cannot make change at a cash register. Lack of academic standards also adversely affects the educators themselves, and 65% of teachers support clear standards to guide their instruction.

The decline in the U.S. education system also has far-reaching consequences for the workforce, as employers rely on employees with standardized skills. It also hurts us in terms of global competitiveness. In 2021, it was estimated that the lack of skills in employees could cost U.S. businesses $1.2 trillion over the next 10 years in lost productivity.

Globally, we rank 11th in education, which further erodes our standing, resulting in weakened innovation and lower economic output. Unsurprisingly, wealthier school districts in the U.S. maintain higher academic standards, which only makes the economic divide greater among high school graduates. In standardized tests, low-income students lag 20% or more behind their wealthier peers.

An often-overlooked consequence of lowering academic standards regards mental health. Clear and high standards, when reached, provide students with achievable goals, which foster motivation and positive self-esteem. Lack of academic standards can lead to students who are disenfranchised, anxious, and disengaged. A 2022 CDC report noted rising mental health issues among teens, partly tied to unclear academic standards.

The impact of lowered expectations for our youth stretches far beyond K-12 schools. Our institutions of higher learning - college and beyond - are also facing a crisis. Overly expensive college tuition, combined with low-skilled degrees, only makes the problem worse. Students amass significant debt in college that can plague them for decades after graduation, affecting their financial freedom. Trade schools are now few and far between, leading to a shortage of skilled workers in traditional careers, such as automotive, electrical, and plumbing. We are facing a societal crisis due to these detrimental changes in our education system.

A less-skilled workforce could actually lead to a shrinking of our GDP growth. In 2023, the World Bank estimated that a 10% drop in educational milestones could reduce our country's GDP by 1-2% annually. Uneven education and skills also fuel division, as workers compete for limited opportunities in the workforce. The basic requirements for employment are likely to increase, not decrease, as we transition to Web3 and AI.

The advancements of technology in medicine are changing the face of healing by the day. Robots now appear in most operating rooms, and AI algorithms are being used by physicians every day. It has even been said that in ten years' time, a physician could face a malpractice lawsuit if they *do not* use AI to help in their patient care. A weakened workforce in medicine, due to declining expectations and standards, is a recipe for professional disaster.

The only way to fight a future where AI replaces those in medicine - as it has in many businesses already - is to *increase* our academic standards, not lower them. We must expect - and demand - more from ourselves and our society. If low-level jobs that have historically employed lower-wage humans are replaced by AI, the uneducated or the undereducated citizen has nowhere to go for alternative employment, if they are unskilled.

Another benefit of *increasing* academic standards is the improved self-esteem that comes with dedication to learning and mastery of new subjects and skills. Grade inflation, where good grades are given despite low performance, weakens the entire class. In fact, a recent study showed that higher college completion rates are largely due to lowering grading standards, rather than improved academic performance.

Faculty surveys at public universities reveal that 47% of tenured professors agree that academic standards have declined, with 48% stating that grade inflation is a serious issue. For example, in California, there is a great discrepancy between the graduating student's high school grades (which are very high and often without merit) and that same student's low proficiency on standardized tests. Currently, in California, only 19% of students meet grade-level expectations. Grade inflation hurts everyone, but especially the students themselves.

Another educational harm arises from prolonged time spent in front of a digital device. This screen time, combined with reduced requirements for learning, harms literacy and cognitive development. We know that the time we spend on most social media platforms does little to help our intellect, and most likely, we are being harmed by this mostly mindless activity.

Our youth is experiencing an epidemic of mental and physical health problems arising from the time spent on these mind-numbing digital activities. A few progressive high schools are now starting to ban cell phones in the classroom, in an attempt to decrease academic distractions.

To have a future with even a glimmer of hope, we must demand more, not less. More from ourselves, more from our education system, and more from our society as a whole.

To have a brighter future, it is time to raise our standards and our voices.

Epilogue
Women in Medicine

Given that this book was written from a female perspective, I felt it was important to research the history of women in medicine, a topic that is not taught in medical school.

In the United States, women physicians in medicine are a relatively recent phenomenon, dating back to 1849, less than 200 years ago at the time of writing this book. As I have written previously, I became a fourth-generation physician in my family, and the only female in my family's lineage to be one.

As you have most likely picked up from my stories in this book, despite my entering class in medical school being 51% female students, female physician mentors were few and far between in my medical training. I was schooled and evaluated all through medical school, internship, and residency by mostly men.

Throughout history, women have traditionally been healers and caregivers, without the title of doctor. While women were typically responsible for medical care within the family, they rarely received a formal medical education or compensation for their knowledge and work. Instead, they used herbal remedies passed down through generations, as well as guidebooks that were published throughout the 1700s.

Beginning in the mid-1800s, cultural shifts led to expanding opportunities for women in medicine as feminism, legal reforms, and societal changes occurred. In 1849, Elizabeth Blackwell became the first female physician in the United States to graduate from Geneva College and Medical School in New York. The next woman to graduate from medical school was Mary Edwards Walker. She graduated from Syracuse Medical College in New York in 1855, six years after Dr. Blackwell.

The first - and only - all-female medical school was Women's Medical College of Pennsylvania (WMCP), established in 1850. It was the first of its kind in the world to exclusively train women as physicians. It faced significant challenges like societal resistance and financial struggles, but graduated many pioneering women doctors over the decades. In 1970, in response to a plethora of other medical schools admitting women into their programs, WMCP began to admit men into its program, eliminating the first and only women-only medical school.

By 1900, 5% of all medical students in the U.S. were female. That percentage didn't change very much over the decades, until it changed drastically in 1972 with the advent of Title IX. Title IX prohibits sex-based discrimination in educational programs. This resulted in a jump in female enrollment in the U.S. medical schools to 25%. By 2010, women made up nearly 50% of all students in medical schools.

But this increase in enrollment of women into medical school has not resulted in parity in the post-doctorate workplace. A 2019 study of physician compensation found that female doctors *still* receive a salary that is 26% less than their male colleagues, for the same job - a shocking statistic. Averaged across all specialties, female physicians earn $121,000 per year less than their male colleagues. This disparity adds up over time, and over a 40-year career, male physicians earn $2,000,000 more than their female counterparts for the same employment.

And, potentially due to the demands of family life, a 2020 study found that female physicians only make up 36% of all practicing physicians. This may indicate that women are completing medical school and residency, but then decide against pursuing a medical career. This contributes to the physician shortage problem. Female physicians are also more likely to be employed part-time. Both of these scenarios have a significant impact on the physician workforce.

To this day, women are also less represented in the more competitive and lucrative specialties, such as neurosurgery and plastic surgery. Challenges for women include harassment in the workplace, as I had experienced in medical school, and underrepresentation in leadership roles. My choice of specialty was definitely informed by my young family and the demands of child rearing. I chose a specialty where *only* 60 hours per week were the norm.

Academic medicine and positions of leadership in universities are another area where there has been a significant divide between male and female physicians. Recent data shows women have made significant strides in academia, but notable disparities remain, especially at senior levels. In the last decade, the percentage of women faculty physicians at medical schools has increased from 38% to 45%. While this is a notable improvement, female physicians only make up 15% of department chairs and hold only 27% of dean positions in the U.S. Progress is evident, but systemic issues persist in achieving equity, especially in the upper echelons of academic medicine.

Women also suffer from a paucity of female mentors in medicine, as I experienced during my training, and the "boy's club" mentality can very easily prevail. Fear of retaliation discourages female trainees from speaking up for themselves, as our careers depend on these faculty evaluations. A 2020 study highlighted that women's perceptions of harassment lead to underreporting due to fears of career repercussions and retaliation. I certainly experienced this during my rotation at the VA with Dr. Harvard. If he had given me the "A" I deserved at the outset, I probably would not have ever reported his harassment and discrimination.

Women are also more likely to question their career choices due to the gender bias they experience. For example, women are less likely to pursue more lucrative specialties due to perceived gender-based hurdles. These include inhospitable work environments and negative assumptions made about family priorities. The impact of these biases and microaggressions against female trainees is substantial.

Sexual discrimination in medicine is a very real thing, even to this day. It is estimated that up to 63% of all women in medicine face gender-based harassment. This includes inappropriate comments, unwanted sexual advances, less time with attendings, and less time in the operating room as compared to our male colleagues. Female trainees are also often stereotyped and judged more harshly on assessments by their peers and supervisors.

Sexism and harassment of women in medicine are strongly linked to negative mental health outcomes. A 2023 Swiss study found that experiencing sexism in medical training leads to increased risks of depression, anxiety, suicidal ideation, and substance use. Female physicians also report higher rates of burnout (37%) as compared to their male colleagues (13%). As stated previously, burnout often leads to depression or even disability claims, further impacting the physician workforce.

Women are also evaluated less on their clinical skills and intellectual acumen. They are judged more critically for their personality traits and even their appearance. In my residency training, I was given the nickname of "Dr. Barbie" because I wore makeup, combed my hair before work, and dressed nicely when not in scrubs.

Female physicians and trainees are often mistaken for nurses or other support staff, as happened to me on the plane, adding to demoralization. In my experience, there is also a clear bias against pregnancy, breastfeeding, and maternity leave, and this can have a significant impact on the choice of specialty a woman chooses. These biases can even cause a woman to no longer pursue medicine as a career.

Regardless of the strides they have made in medicine, female physicians face significant challenges related to several hurdles. At the top of the list - as it was for me - was the concept of work-life balance. As a physician in training and mother of two young children, the demands on my time, away from my medical practice, were significant.

At times, it felt like a daily struggle between caring for my family and caring for my patients. While this could be said of many different professions, the irony of caring for the sick or unwell is that it does not translate into sick time for physicians themselves. Somehow, in the zeitgeist of medicine, doctors are not supposed to call in sick. Ever. Superhuman health and complete dedication to your career are the norm, and what is expected of you.

Medicine has been called a "jealous mistress," and at times in my training and career, I felt that sentiment deeply. Oftentimes, if I was at work, I was thinking of home and my children. And when at home, I thought about work and my patients. A never-ending mental, emotional, and physical seesaw that I did my best to balance, but oftentimes left me feeling inept at both.

Would my training and career in medicine have been easier if I didn't have children, or even a spouse? Unequivocally yes. Would I do things differently if given the choice to redo my medical career without a family? Absolutely not. Children have a way of humbling you on par with losing a patient. And, in my opinion and experience, children enrich your life in a way a medical career never could.

My children made me a better doctor, and being a doctor helped me be a better mother.

Namaste.

About the Author

Liz **Casper** is an accomplished artist, author, and former fourth-generation physician from the Pacific Northwest. In her second book, *Learning to Heal*, Liz chronicles her journey through medicine, shaped by science and art. Through honest, raw, and captivating storytelling, Liz shares with her readers her experience as she completed medical school and residency; stories from her career as a private practice physician; and her journey as a patient herself, battling cancer.

Learning to Heal is a tribute to the medical profession and the exceptional commitment and resilience one must demonstrate to become a physician. Liz's witty prose and sardonic humor add insight and levity to the grueling path one must take in the pursuit of an allopathic medical doctorate. She entertains and educates her readers with captivating storytelling. Physicians and lay people alike will enjoy her unique perspective on the pursuit of an M.D. degree and her experience as a woman in medicine.

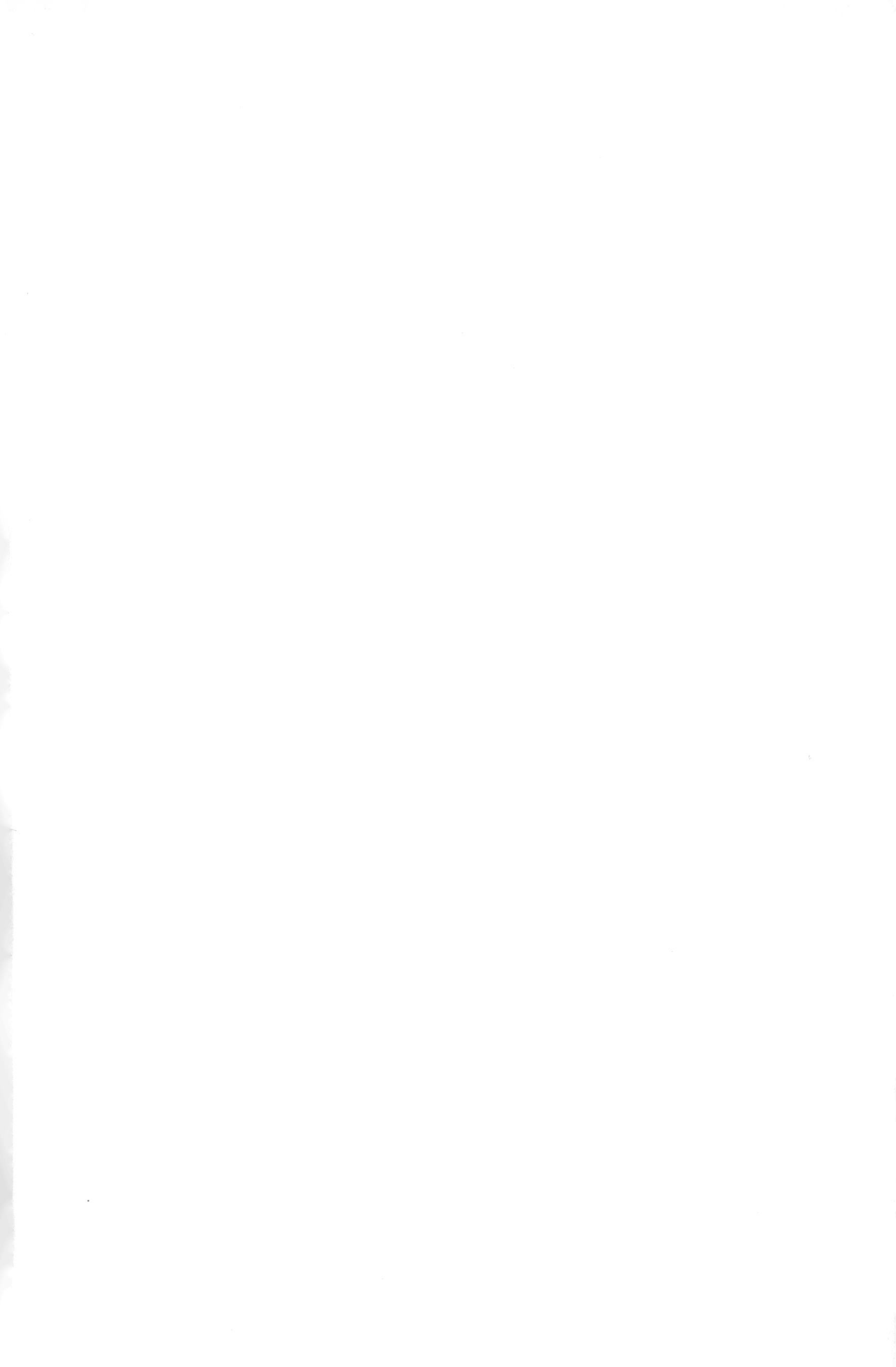